AF292681

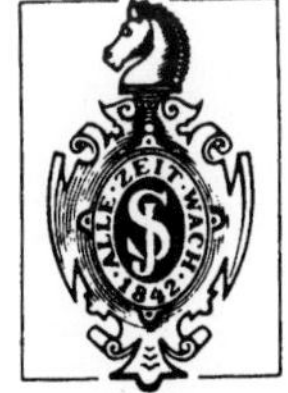

U. Gresser, N. Zöllner (Eds.)

Urate Deposition in Man and its Clinical Consequences

With Contributions by
R. A. De Abreu, G. van den Berghe, G. Calabrese, D. J. McCarty,
B. T. Emmerson, B. Gathof, M. Gonella, U. Gresser, W. Gröbner,
I. Kamilli, W. Löffler, W. Mohr, G. Nuki, D. Perrett, J. G. Puig, F. Roch-
Ramel, M. Schattenkirchner, K. L. Schmidt, J. T. Scott, H. A. Simmonds,
O. Sperling, R. Terkeltaub, R. W. E. Watts, H. F. Woods, N. Zöllner

With 53 Figures and 26 Tables

Springer-Verlag
Berlin Heidelberg New York London Paris Tokyo
Hong Kong Barcelona Budapest

Privatdozentin Dr. Ursula Gresser
Professor Dr. Nepomuk Zöllner
Medizinische Poliklinik der Universität München
Pettenkoferstraße 8 a, W-8000 München 2

ISBN-13:978-3-642-84493-5   e-ISBN-13:978-3-642-84491-1
DOI: 10.1007/978-3-642-84491-1

2127/3335-543210 – Printed on acid-free paper

List of Contributors

Prof. Dr. R. A. De Abreu
Academisch Ziekenhuis Nijmegen, Sint-Radboudziekenhuis,
Postbus 9101, NL-6500 HB Nijmegen

Prof. Dr. G. van den Berghe
International Institute of Cellular and Molecular Pathology, UCL 7539,
Avenue Hippocrate 75, B-1200 Bruxelles

Dr. G. Calabrese
Servizio di Nefrologia e Dialisi, Ente Ospedaliero, I-15033 Casale Monferrato (Al)

Prof. Dr. D. J. McCarty
Medical College of Wisconsin, 8700 W. Wisconsin Ave., Milwaukee Wi.
53226, USA

Prof. Dr. B. T. Emmerson
University of Queensland, Department of Medicine, Princess Alexandra
Hospital, Brisbane, Queensland, Australia 4102

Dr. B. Gathof
Medizinische Poliklinik der Universität München, Pettenkoferstr. 8a,
 D-8000 München 2

Prof. Dr. M. Gonella
Servizio di Nefrologia e Dialisi, Ente Ospedaliero, I-15033 Casale Monferrato

Priv.-Doz. Dr. Ursula Gresser
Medizinische Poliklinik der Universität München, Pettenkoferstr. 8a,
 D-8000 München 2

Prof. Dr. W. Gröbner
Kreiskrankenhaus Balingen, Tübinger Str. 30, D-7460 Balingen

Dr. I. Kamilli
Medizinische Poliklinik der Universität München, Pettenkoferstr. 8 a,
 D-8000 München 2

Priv.-Doz. Dr. W. Löffler
Städt. Krankenhaus M-Bogenhausen, Englschalkinger-Str. 27, D-8000 München 81

Prof. Dr. W. Mohr
Abteilung Pathologie der Universität Ulm,
Albert-Einstein-Allee 11, D-7900 Ulm

Prof. Dr. G. Nuki
Rheumatic Diseases Unit, Northern General Hospital, Ferry Road, Edinburgh
EH5 2DQ, Großbritannien

Dr. D. Perrett
Dept. of Medicine, St. Bartholomew's Hospital, London EC 1 A 7 BE, Great
Britain

Prof. Dr. J. G. Puig
Hospital "La Paz" Costa Brava 23 30 D, E-28034 Madrid

Prof. Dr. F. Roch-Ramel
Institut de Pharmacologie et de Toxicologie de l'Université de Lausanne,
Rue de Bugnon 27, CH-1005 Lausanne

Prof. Dr. M. Schattenkirchner
Medizinische Poliklinik der Universität München, Pettenkoferstraße 8 a,
D-8000 München 2

Prof. Dr. K. Schmidt
Klinik für Physikalische Medizin, Balneologie und Rheumatologie am
Klinikum der Justus-Liebig-Universität Gießen Bad Nauheim, Ludwigstr.
37–39, D-6350 Bad Nauheim

Prof. Dr. J. T. Scott
Charing Cross Hospital, Department of Rheumatology, Fulham Palace Road,
Hammersmith, London W6 8RF, Großbritannien

Prof. Dr. H. A. Simmonds
Clinical Science Laboratories, Guy's Tower (17th and 18th Floors), Guy's
Hospital, London Bridge, SE1 9RT, Großbritannien

Prof. Dr. O. Sperling
Beilinson Medical Center, School of Medicine, Tel-Aviv University,
49 100 Petah-Tiqva, Israel

Prof. Dr. R. Terkeltaub
Rheum. Section, V. A. Medical Center, III-K, 3350 La Jolla Village Drive,
San Diego, CA 92 161, USA

Prof. Dr. R. W. E. Watts
14, Holly Lodge Gardens, Highgate, London N6 6AA, Großbritannien

Prof. Dr. H. F. Woods
The University of Sheffield, Department of Medicine and Pharmacology,
Royal Hallamshire Hospital, Glossop Road, Sheffield S10 2JF, Großbritan-
nien

Prof. Dr. N. Zöllner
Medizinische Poliklinik der Universität München, Pettenkoferstr. 8 a,
 D-8000 München 2

Contents

1

The Study of Inborn Errors of Metabolism – 40 Years of Experience at the Poliklinik of the University of Munich

N. ZÖLLNER

Introduction

Every one of us larows of patients with gout in whom tophi were found in the vicinity of joints which had never experienced a gouty attack. We have heard of their painless growth and consequent articular malfunction. There are old reports in the literature describing urate needles in articular cartilage of patients with chronic renal insufficiency, and those of us who are close to a department of orthopedics have seen menisci or heads of femur removed because of coxarthrosis, in which in connection with hyperuricemia the joint surface was covered by a white substance which was murexide positive.

Thirty years ago I published a review entitled "Moderne Gichtprobleme, Ätiologie, Pathogenese, Klinik" [1]. Several pages were taken to describe cases of asymptomatic consequences of hyperuricemia, particularly subcutaneous tophi not originating from a joint, clinically inapparent tophi of the bones, asymptomatic tophi of the bursae, and even tophi at the rim of the cornea and in the episclera. In the same review I mentioned reports on a case of subluxation of the first cervical vertebra and a case of paraplegia as a complication of gout. Obviously, the case histories existed, but the problem was not recognized. Meanwhile, we have seen several patients with carpal tunnel syndrome (as have others), one of them reported in the German literature [2], and two patients with paraplegia, one of them described on a poster [3].

Those early observations clearly demonstrated the possibility of urate precipitation in certain tissues of hyperuricemic patients. Of course, there are a number of questions which had been posed then, although they remain unanswered. Let us assume that research into the pathogenesis of the gouty attack, so brilliantly begun by McCarty and Hollander, the advent of new therapeutic possibilities, and the advances in purine research attracted all eyes and postponed preoccupation with an issue of seemingly minor clinical importance. Finally, the Framingham study and other similar endeavors related only the probability of gouty attacks and renal colics to the degree of hyperuricemia, overlooking the well-known other manifestations of gout. Therefore, around that time we all commenced evaluating the therapy of hyperuricemia from its capacity to prevent attacks, which can easily be measured,

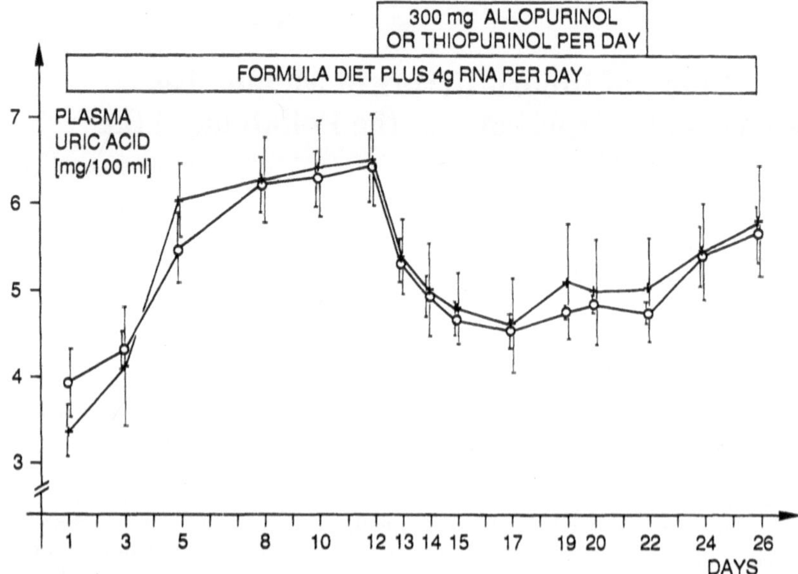

Fig. 1. Effects of allopurinol and of a similar substance on uric acid plasma levels in an experiment controlled by a formula diet

and no longer tried to take painless urate depositions into account. Some of us went so far as to say that hyperuricemia of whatever degree would not merit therapy unless the patient had experienced several attacks of gout or renal colic.

While preparing the relevant chapter for our new book on hyperuricemia and gout [4], it became obvious that urate deposition was a neglected field of uric acid research. Three generous sponsors (Henning, Janssen, Wellcome) enabled us to contact known specialists from all over the world. Most of those to whom I wrote immediately agreed that a discussion of the subject would be timely and offered to speak or to discuss.

My coworkers asked me not to stop my introduction at this point but to review the 40 years of research in purine metabolism at the Medizinische Poliklinik of the University of Munich.

When I graduated from Medical School, World War II was in its last stages. At the end of the war, people in Germany were extremely poor. Nobody had enough to eat; everybody felt cold, very cold; and there was no access to modern and useful information except in the "America houses." In 1948, I had the fortune to obtain a scholarship to Tufts University in Boston. I had published a few papers on the free electrophoresis of plasma proteins.

When I arrived in Boston, exactly 42 years and 1 week ago, my professor Siegfried Thannhauser told me that his laboratory would not work on proteins

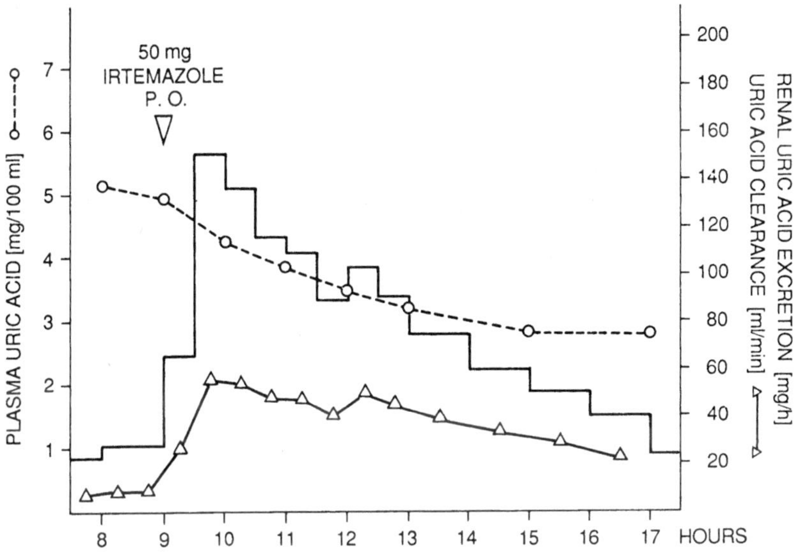

Fig. 2. Effect of a single dose of 50 mg irtemazole on uric acid excretion, uric acid level in plasma, and uric acid clearance in healthy volunteers

but on the metabolism of nucleic acids and lipids. That first interview, no longer than 10 min, directed the research work of my life. I spent all my days and part of my nights in the laboratory, working on acetalphosphatides and on the enzymatic degradation of RNA. I had very little time for clinical work. I think that a good scientist may become a good doctor, while a good doctor has much less of a chance to become a good scientist.

When I returned from the USA, due to the generosity of my then chief and now friend Walter Seitz I obtained sufficient laboratory space, about 100 square yards. Also, I established a small outpatient clinic for metabolic diseases. It turned out that this combination was and remained the main stay of the work. We always worked on hyperlipidemias and disorders of purine metabolism, more or less in parallel. This was of tremendous value because the methods and tools are quite similar in both fields, sharing enzymatic analysis, various types of chromatography, formula diets, tissue cell cultures, and molecular genetics. Those in the group working on purines could profit from the experiences of those working on lipids and vice versa. Of course, at first the work was mainly clinical, and evaluations of therapeutic possibilities were carried out. Every possibly uricosuric substance within reach was studied, I should guess about 25 in all.

Later, Wellcome was kind enough to ask us for the first German study on allopurinol. Other firms have requested investigations of substances similiar

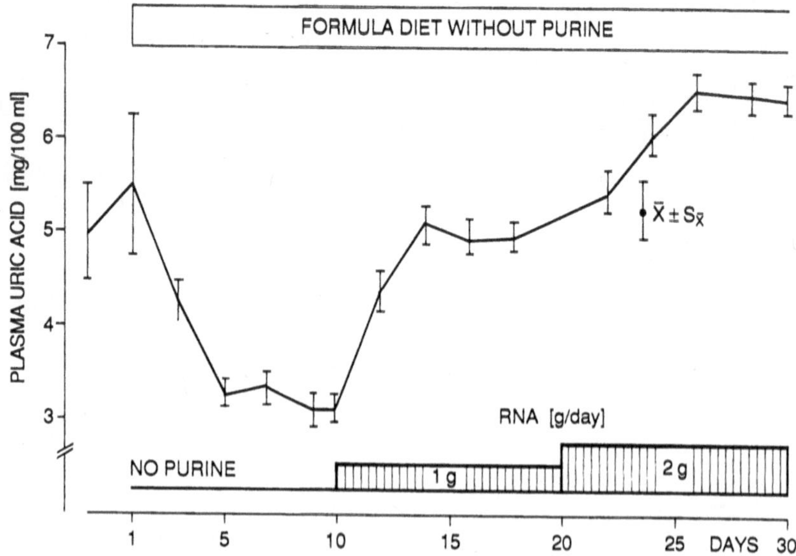

Fig. 3. Uric acid plasma levels on a purine-free formula diet, supplemented stepwise with RNA

to allopurinol (Fig. 1), but none proved to be as good. The most recent project is a new uricosuric drug, irtemazole (Fig. 2).

All this work was supported greatly by a new enzymatic method for the determination of uric acid [5]; it was much better than the old Folin method, even when the latter was combined with enzymatic oxidation of uric acid, and it still is better than the other new method in which the enzymatic degradation is combined with a color reaction, which is not entirely specific. So the old method is still used for reference in cases of doubt.

My main coworker at that time was Katharina Kirsch, who now works with Isselbacher in Boston, while Günther Wolfram and Christiane Keller worked on lipids. Around that time Wolfgang Gröbner joined us, went away to Durham to work with Kelley and Holmes, and came back with new techniques and new ideas. We were interested in why most American authors claimed that diet is of no use in the therapy of gout (except Goodman and Yü, who found that with a proper diet one could lower plasma urate levels by 1.2 mg/dl). A "lipid friendship" with E. H. Ahrens, Jr., led to the idea of developing a formula diet for the study of uric acid. A basic formula containing nearly no purines which could be supplemented by defined purine sources was created. First, it was established that on a no purine diet, plasma uric acid and renal uric acid excretion levels dropped much more than predicted (Fig. 3). We also found, and this was very interesting, that in hyperuricemic members of families suffering from gout, plasma uric acid concentration

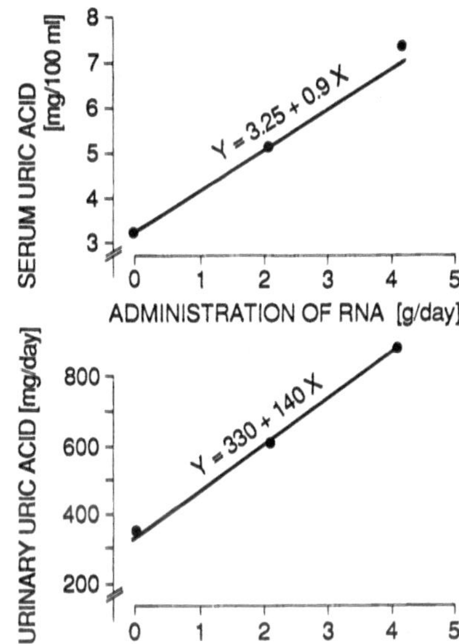

Fig. 4. Influence of graded addition of RNA to a purine-free formula diet on plasma levels and urinary excretion of uric acid

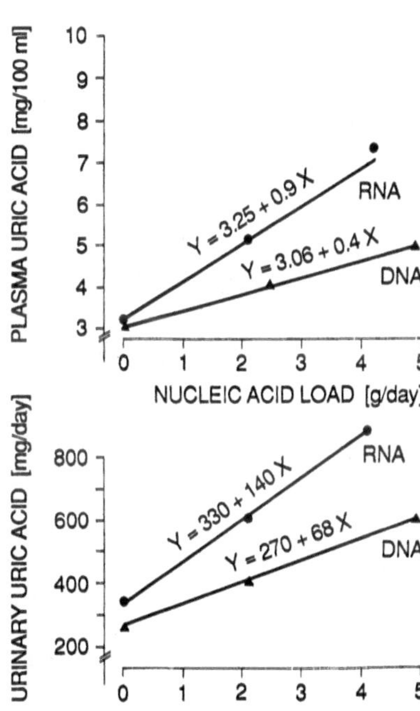

Fig. 5. Differing influences of graded additions of RNA or DNA to a purine-free formula diet on plasma levels and urinary excretion of uric acid

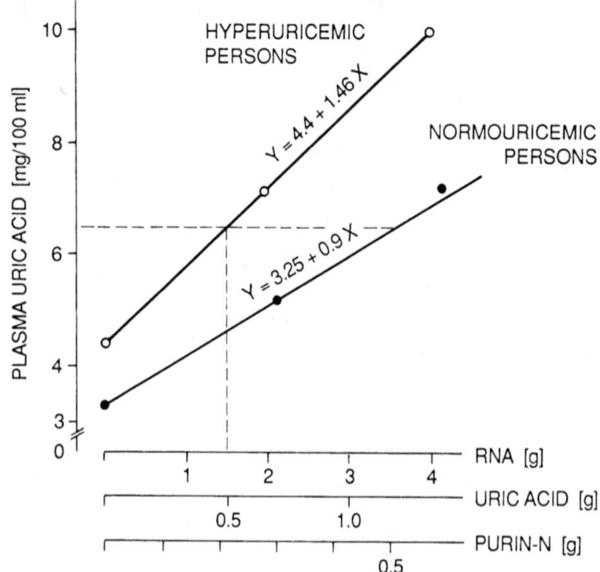

Fig. 6. Influence of graded additions of RNA to a purine-free formula diet on uric acid plasma levels of persons who were normouricemic or greatly hyperuricemic on average diets before the experiment. (Some of the hyperuricemic probands had a positive family history for gout)

dropped as well. This provided the explanation why in Europe, i. e., Norway, Federal Republic of Germany, and France, during World War II gout disappeared. It was then discovered that graded additions of RNA led to a linear increase of plasma uric acid and uric acid excretion (Fig. 4); nothing very new. We could also establish that the source of the dietary purine was of the utmost importance, the effect of RNA on uric acid levels was more than twice that DNA (Fig. 5), purine mononucleotides were quantitively taken up from the gut. All these results show the limited usefulness of food tables which give purine values.

Finally, we found (and most of this work has been done by Anton Griebsch, affectionately called "Sir Anthony", and Wolfgang Gröbner) that the addition of purine sources to the formula diet led in patients with gout (or their hyperuricemia relatives) to a much steeper increase in plasma uric acid levels than in normal controls (Fig. 6), while the excretion of uric acid by the kidney was the same in both groups. This, of course, proves that an excretion defect is the reason for hyperuricemia in nearly all cases of gout (Fig. 7). Formula diets could be used to demonstrate that allopurinol acts preferentially on dietary purine (Fig. 8) and that dietary purines in humans enter the purine metabolism to a negligible degree, a conclusion which was later

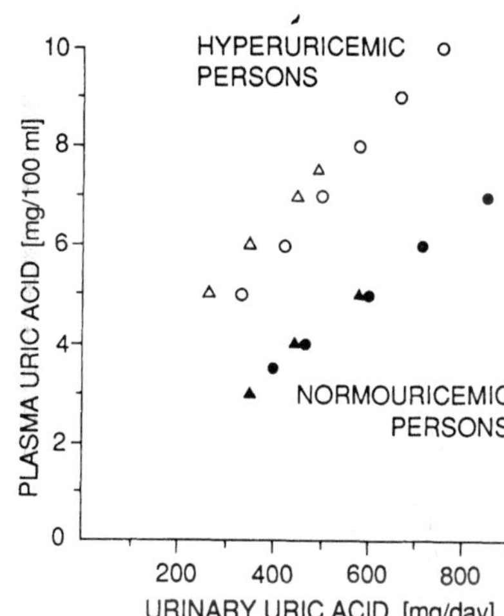

Fig. 7. Correlation between plasma uric acid level and uric acid excretion in subjects described in Fig. 6

proven by Werner Löffler, using a combination of isotope research and formula diet. Finally, Wolfgang Gröbner showed that the effects of allopurinol on pyrimidine metabolism are greatly influenced by dietary purines.

Parallel to that work, we continued searching for special cases. Wolfgang Gröbner identified our first case of hypoxanthine-guanine phosphoribosyl-transferase (HGPRT) deficiency, a gentleman who still comes to our service.

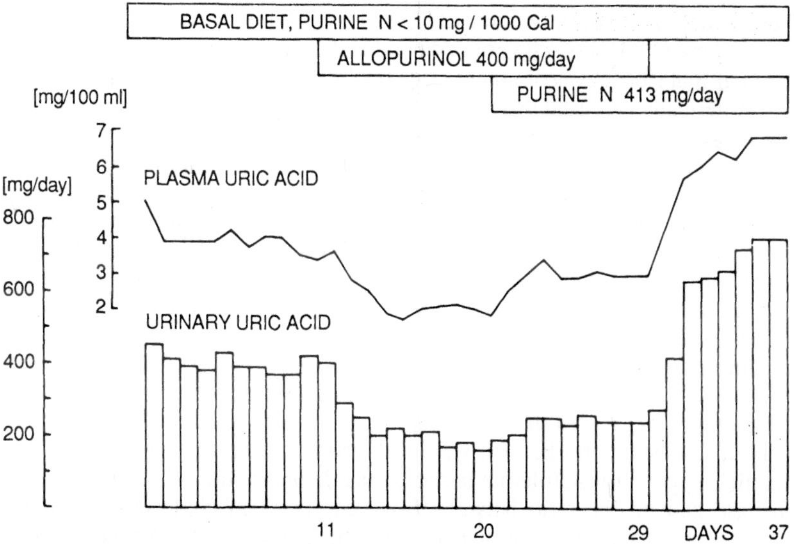

Fig. 8. Influence of allopurinol on endogenous and exogenous uric acid

Gröbner also carried out a number of studies on this patient's enzyme isolated from erythrocytes and fibroblast cultures. Finally, the enzyme was characterized by Bill Kelley; it is now known in the literature as HGPRT Munich. If one looks carefully, HGPRT deficiencies are not very rare. We have seen a number of cases in the intervening years without searching too hard for them.

By 1980, Wolfgang Gröbner had left, I had become chairholding full professor (1973), and Sebastian Reiter had taken over the purine laboratory. At that time, we already had received considerable assistance from our British colleagues, Anne Simmonds, who helped to acquire modern methodology and in whose laboratory Löffler and Reiter were guests, Richard Watts, a former fellow of J. Seegmiller, who advised us, and Francis Woods, a former coworker of Sir Hans Krebs and now professor of medicine in Sheffield who thoroughly questioned some of our clinical concepts, not to forget Tom Scott to whom we own many interesting discussions, and again Anne Simmonds together with Cameron whose ideas on gouty nephropathy we cannot share.

In the course of the years I found that every fellow is a person of his own. One can force people to do work they do not like, but not without loss of intensity, intelligence, and devotion. Our definition of teamwork reads: "Everybody does what he likes, nobody does what the chief thinks he should do, but all cooperate."

Reiter decided to work on the metabolism of allopurinol and on the differences between xanthine oxidase and aldehyde dehydrogenase. Together with Anne Simmonds he studied xanthinuric patients.

A little later we became interested in AMP deaminase deficiency, because we had diagnosed the first German sufferer. With the aid of faulty reasoning I decided that the administration of ribose should help my patient, much to the astonishment of Reiter who pointed out that the American literature contained a report that ribose was of no use. Again with faulty reasoning I told him that the Americans had used doses which were much too low and that we should try it; we were successful. Our patient, an ardent skier who had repeatedly lain with painful cramps in the middle of a slope, could ski freely when he drank the ribose solutions his pharmacist supplied him with. My theory why ribose should work was wrong, but ribose still works; the most recent result from our laboratory shows that ribose is also effective in McArdle's disease. By that time, Reiter and Löffler had left us to follow their respective careers, but not before helping Manfred Gross who is now at Duke's and works with Ed Holmes on experiments of ribose metabolism.

Our collection of patients with gout never became too large because the rheumatologists also laid claim to them. Our lipid department had no such competitor, and a wealth of material could be accumulated. Following the lead of Goldstein and Brown, we developed comparatively simple tests for familial hypercholesterolemia based on the determination of HMG-CoA reductase and on the ratio between free and esterified cholesterol in tissue cultures, a test which discriminated 100% [6]. The very large patient material which accumulated proved to be of particular benefit. One family did not fit

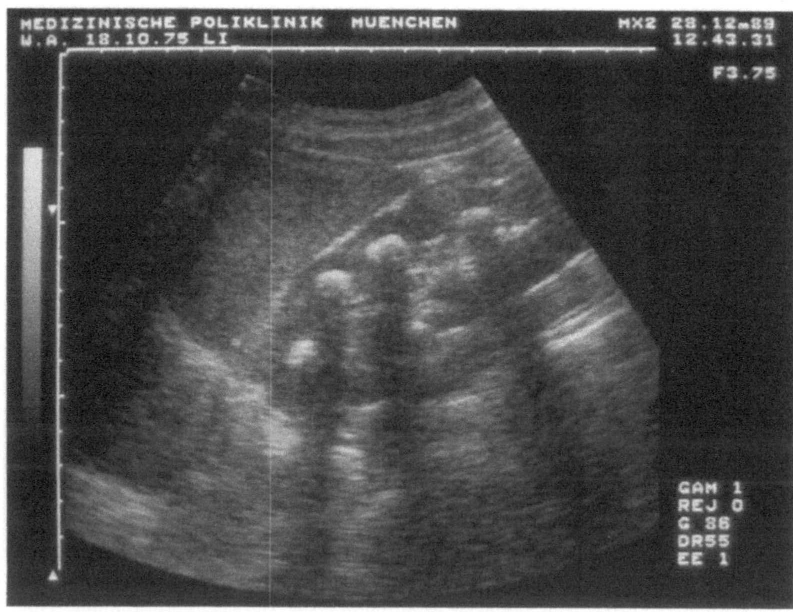

Fig. 9. Sonogram of a kidney of one of the twins with APRT deficiency showing multiple stones

the accepted theories and forced us to assume that along with all the known defects leading to hypercholesterolemia, there are a few more, still unidentified (6a). Dr. Harders-Spengel isolated the normal receptor and the defective receptor from human liver and published the results in the *Proceedings of the National Academy of Science* (6b). Most important was the introduction of molecular genetics into the work on hyperlipidemias by Dr. Schuster, who established, with the use of several restriction enzymes, that patients with familial hypercholesterolemia are not genetically homogenous; approximately 10 of the more than 30 known variants of this disease are found in Munich (6c). After discovering the point mutation in apo B-100, Schuster and his colleague Rauh identified cases among our patients (6d).

When Reiter left, Ursula Gresser became the new head of the purine laboratory. Concurrently, two important things happened. After a long interim a new uricosuric drug was offered for study [7–9], and a colleague from urology had asked me to help him with twins with APRT deficiency (Fig. 9). I will not go into the work on irtemazole because I have mentioned it before, but I should like to comment briefly on the APRT (Adenine-phosphoribosyl-transferase) deficient twins [10]. They are, as far as I know, the only probands in Germany. The results of analyses in molecular genetics look most interesting but are as yet unpublished.

The directions of purine research have changed in this laboratory as well as all over the world. At present, one must be careful to continue working on purine metabolism and not to deviate too much, e. g., to molecular genetics. Insights into the mechanisms and pathogenesis of disease must remain our aim [11, 12]. Forty years of purine research proved that one must stay with a subject in order to produce useful results, while interests, ideas, methods, and tools change continuously.

References

1. Zöllner N (1960) Moderne Gichtprobleme, Ätiologie, Pathogenese, Klinik. In: Heilmeyer L, Schoen R, de Rudder B (Hrsg) Ergebnisse der Inneren Medizin und Kinderheilkunde N.F. 14: 321–389
2. Walther B, Bauer H, Gröbner W, Zöllner N (1982) Karpaltunnelsyndrom bei Gicht. DMW 107: 942–944
3. Wallmüller-Strycker A, Walther B, Gröbner W, Zöllner N (1980) Zwei seltene neurologische Komplikationen bei Gicht. Vortr. 19. Tagung Dt. Ges. Rheumatologie 30. 9.–4.10.1980, Konstanz
4. Zöllner N (1990) Hyperurikämie, Gicht und andere Störungen des Purinhaushalts. Springer, Berlin Heidelberg New York
5. Zöllner N (1963) Eine einfache Modifikation der Harnsäurebestimmung. Normalwerte in der deutschen Bevölkerung. Z Klin Chem 1: 178–182
6. Spengel FA, Harders-Spengel KM, Keller CHF, Wieczorek A, Wolfram G, Zöllner N (1982) Use of Fibroblast Culture to Diagnose and Genotype Familial Hypercholesterolaemia. Ann Nutr Metab 26: 240–247
6a. Harders-Spengel K, Wood CB, Thompson GR, Myant NB, Soutar AK (1982) Difference in saturable binding of low-density-lipoprotein to liver membrane from normocholesterolemic subjects and patients with heterozygous familial hypercholesterolemia. Proc Natl Acad USA 79: 6355–6359
6b. Keller C, Harders-Spengel K, Spengel F, Wieczorek A, Wolfram G, Zöllner N (1981) Serum cholesterol levels in patients with familial hypercholesterolemia confirmed by tissue culture. Atherosclerosis 39: 51–59
6c. Schuster H, Stiefenhofer B, Wolfram G, Keller C, Humphries S, Huber A, Zöllner N (1989) 4 DNA polymorphisms in the LDL-receptor gene and their use in diagnosis of FH. Hum Genet 82 (I): 69–72
6d. Schuster H, Rauh G, Kormann B, Hepp T, Humphries S, Keller C, Wolfram G, Zöllner N (1990) Familial defective apolipoprotein B-100: Comparison with familial hypercholesterolemia in 18 cases detected in Munich. Arteriosclerosis 10, 4: 577–581
7. Gresser U, Zöllner N (1989) Uricosuric Effect of Irtemazole in Healthy Subjects. Klin Wochenschr 67: 971–975
8. Kamilli I, Gresser U, Pellkofer T, Löffler W and Zöllner N (1989) Uricosuric Effect of Irtemazole in Hyperuricemic Patients without and with Renal Insufficiency. Z Rheumatol 48: 307–312
9. Gresser U, Kamilli I, Kronawitter U and Zöllner N (1990) Uricosuric Effect of Different Doses of Irtemazole in Normouricaemic Subjects. Eur J Clin Pharmacol 38: 489–491

10. Zöllner N and Gresser U (1990) Nephrolithiasis in Twins with APRT-deficiency. Stones as a Marker of an Inborn Error of Metabolism. Imaging/Bildgebung 57: 64–66
11. Zöllner N, Gresser U and Walter-Sack I (1990) Deficient benzbromarone elimination: a familial disorder? Klin Wochenschr 68: 101
12. Gresser U, Gathof B and Zöllner N (1990) Uric Acid Levels in Southern Germany 1989. A Comparison with Studies from 1962, 1971 and 1984. Klin Wochenschr 68: 1222–1228

Questions and Comments Raised for Discussion

G. VAN DEN BERGHE

Was glycogen concentration measured in the muscle of patients with AMP deaminase deficiency, and was it elevated?

The observation that ribose acts both in AMP deaminase deficiency and in McArdle's disease may suggest that it circumvenes a common block in both disorders. If one hypothesizes that ribose acts by entering (more rapidly than glucose?) the glycolytic pathway at the level of fructose-6-phosphate after passing through the pentose phosphate shunt, this block might be located higher up in the glycolytic pathway or in the glycogenolytic pathway. If the latter is the case, one might expect an accumulation of glycogen. This would indicate that AMP deaminase results, for example, in the accumulation of an inhibitor of glycogen degradation.

2

The Enigma of Urate Deposition

H. F. Woods

The deposition of urate in the form of a tophus is a characteristic feature of gout. The tophus comprises a mass of urate crystals surrounded by acute inflammatory cells, with an outer layer of giant cells and epithelial cells. Larger deposits – nodules – are made up of large masses of urate (hydrated monosodium urate) together with acute inflammatory cells and giant cells. Calcium salts are commonly included along with fat, protein and polysaccharides. The processes that lead up to the deposition of urate in tissues appear, at first consideration, simple. The solubility of monosodium urate in human plasma is saturated at 7 mg/dl (Seegmiller 1965). At concentrations around or above 7 mg/dl, the urate would be expected to precipitate out to form tophi.

Support for this thesis comes from clinical observations such as those which show that the rate of tophus formation is related to the extent and duration of an elevated serum urate concentration (Gutman 1973), and there is a link between the severity of gout and the degree of renal damage in patients with established gout (Talbott and Terplan 1960). There is also a relationship between the serum urate concentration and the prevalence of acute gouty arthritis and urinary tract stones (Woods 1990).

However, this thesis is too simplistic for three reasons. Firstly, the fact that the serum urate concentration is at or about saturation point in human plasma does not of necessity mean that urate will be deposited out of solution. Secondly, the deposition of urate as tophi does not occur in all patients who have an elevated plasma urate concentration. Thirdly, urate deposition follows a non-uniform anatomical pattern, suggesting that tissue or "environmental" factors may be involved in the initiation or regulation of deposition.

The solubility of urate in plasma is a matter for discussion. Supersaturated solutions have been documented in patients following cytotoxic chemotherapy (Gold and Fritz 1957). These were stable, and although in many cases we cannot be certain that microscopic, subclinical tophi are not present, it is a matter of clinical observation that not all patients with grossly elevated plasma urate concentrations develop tophi or other manifestations of urate deposition. The factors leading to the stability of supersaturated plasma urate solutions have been the subject of debate (Morris 1958; Kovarsky et al. 1979), and we remain ignorant as far as the factors which initiate urate deposition are concerned.

The second point is illustrated by the work of Gutman (1973) who showed that 10 years after a first attack of gout half of the patients were without tophi.

Tophi occur frequently in connective tissue such as tendons, cartilage and synovial membrane. Some anatomical sites are commonly affected, such as the helix of the ear and the peripheral joints, while others like the myocardium, blood vessels and muscles are only rarely involved. These facts taken together with the non-uniform distribution of urate deposits in severe tophaceous gout strongly suggests that tissue-related factors influence urate deposition.

The natural history of gout has been altered by the introduction of effective drugs (Yu 1974). In particular, the incidence of tophaceous gout has fallen. This symposium is concerned with the subject of urate deposition, a process which is not fully understood. Better understanding could further improve the efficacy of therapy, particularly in "resistant" cases.

References

1. Gold GL and Fritz RD (1957) Hyperuricaemia associated with the treatment of acute leukaemia. Ann Intern Med 47: 428–434
2. Glutman AB (1973) The past four decades of progress in the knowledge of gout, with an assessment of the present status. Arthritis Rheum 16: 431–435
3. Kovarsky J, Holmes E, and Kelley WN (1979) Absence of significant urate binding to plasma proteins. J Lab Clin Med 93: 85–91
4. Morris JE (1958) The transport of uric acid in serum. Am J Med Sci 235: 43–49
5. Seegmiller JE (1965) The acute attack of gouty arthritis. Arthritis Rheum 8: 714–723
6. Talbott JH and Terplan KL (1960) The kidney in gout. Medicine 39: 405–467
7. Woods HF (1990) Wann behandelt man die Hyperurikamie? In: Zöllner N (Hrsg) Hyperurikamie, Gicht und andere Störungen des Purinhaushalts. Springer-Verlag, Berlin Heidelberg New York, pp 253–259
8. Yu TF (1974) Milestones in the treatment of gout. Am J Med 56: 676–685

Questions and Comments Raised for Discussion

D. J. McCarty

Controversy regarding which comes first in the development of a gouty tophus, sodium urate crystal deposition or focal necrosis was at the turn of the century seemingly resolved by the demonstration of tissue necrosis after injection of synthetic crystals into man and rabbit.

Factors possibly related to localization of crystal deposits include: (1) temperature; (2) local pH; (3) differential tissue clearance rates of water and urate anion or local dehydration; (4) avascularity (implicates a proteoglycan aggregate effect on solubility or glycosaminoglycan effects as a cation exchanger); (5) local nucleating agents (calcium phosphate crystals, colloidal urate, lead urate, pre-existing tissue damage, trauma-induced necrosis, aging changes). Cartilage per se appears to favor sodium urate crystal nucleation and growth. The recent demonstration of acini composed of tissue macrophages surrounding crystal-free necrotic foci again raises the question of whether the crystal deposition is a secondary phenomenon.

Tophus enlargement requires hard tissue removal to create new space. This may be accomplished by the ability of endocytosed crystals stimulating the synthesis and secretion of proteases, including collagenase, stromelysin and gelatinase from fibroblasts, macrophages, synovial cells or chondrocytes. Crystal-stimulated phospholipase A_1 activity also generates arachidonic acid which is converted to PGE_2 by cyclo-oxygenase.

Studies relating to the mechanism of tophus development may lead to a better understanding of the metabolic associates of gout such as hypertension, obesity, hyperlipidemia and atherosclerosis.

Precipitation and Deposition of Monosodium Urate Monohydrate Crystals in Tissues

D. J. McCarty

Gout (L. *gutta* – a drop) is defined here as the presence of monosodium urate monohydrate (MSU) crystals in human tissues. MSU needles or spheres are a constant feature of symptomatic gouty arthritis, whether this is due to inflammation in the acute attack or to destructive arthropathy in tophaceous gout [1]. Hyperuricemia, defined as a serum urate level greater than 7.0 mg/dl, is a very frequent, but not indispensable, requirement for MSU crystal deposition. There are multiple pathways to hyperuricemia, but MSU crystals are the final common pathway of gout. The crystals most commonly deposit in articular tissues such as synovium, cartilage, and bone, in skin, and in the pyramids of the kidney [2]. MSU deposition favors the acral, cooler parts of the body such as the pinnae of the ears, tips of the olecranon, distal interphalangeal (DIP) joints (especially Heberden's nodes) of the fingers, and the toe joints, especially the IP and metatarsal-phalangeal (MTP) joints of the great toe. The solubility of MSU at 30°C is only 4 mg/dl vs 7 mg/dl at 37°C [3].

Why don't all hyperuricemic individuals deposit MSU crystals in their feet? Why don't all of us develop such deposits? Why doesn't the entire hyperuricemic extracellular fluid compartment crystallize from a single seed crystal? Why is MSU crystal deposition focal at all? Although much is known about both MSU crystals and purine metabolism and gout has become perhaps the most successfully treated metabolic disease in medicine, we cannot answer these questions which have been regarded as pivotal ever since A. B. Garrod demonstrated an excess of uric acid in the serum of most patients with gout in 1876 [4].

Historical Review

Much speculation and experimentation followed Garrod's observation. Histology was the cutting edge of medical science in the late nineteenth century, and it was applied vigorously to the study of tophi and crystal-encrusted tissues of both patients and experimental animals. The observation of MSU crystal phagocytosis by polymorphonuclear and mononuclear leukocytes in fresh skin tophi by the Viennese dermatologist Gustave Riehl [5] was succeeded by the injection of synthetic MSU needle-shaped crystals subcutaneously into rabbits by Wilhelm His, Jr., and Max Freudweiler [6].

On two occasions injections were made into Freudweiler. An inflammatory reaction invariably followed each injection, with gradual evolution of a mass of crystals walled off by freshly proliferated fibroblasts and multinucleated giant cells. Focal necrosis occurred initially in the tissue contacted by the injected crystals. Such granulomatous lesions met the histomorphometric criteria which the authors had established for human skin tophi. Freudweiler, back home in Zurich, produced hyperuricemia in chickens by ureteral ligation [7]. He injected uric acid or MSU crystals or caused local burn necrosis at various times before ligation. He found that most crystal deposition occurred in the viscera, especially the pericardial sac, and that the inflamed tissue around the injected crystals attracted fresh MSU crystal deposits, whereas necrotic tissue did not.

These findings seemed to settle what was apparently a raging controversy over the pathogenesis of the gouty tophus. These theories as summarized by Freudweiler [6] generally regarded MSU crystal deposition as an epiphenomenon. Theories of primary local tissue devitalization and necrosis which then favored crystal deposition implicated trauma (Fagge), focal necrosis (Ebstein), an "unknown ferment" (V. Norden), "gouty matter" (Klemperer), or a "toxic affinity for uric acid" (Holland, Parkes, Barclay). As the injected MSU crystals had caused tissue necrosis and as necrotic foci caused by crystals or by a burn failed to cause MSU crystal deposition in hyperuricemic chickens, Freudweiler's data supported the notion that crystal formation per se was the primary event in the development of a tophus. He criticized the techniques used by Ebstein, V. Norden, and Klemperer, who had found necrotic tissue foci devoid of MSU crystals in both patients and experimental animals. These workers had apparently used aqueous fixtives, thought by His and Freudweiler to have dissolved the crystals from the necrotic foci.

It is worthwhile to consider what was known about gout in 1900 (reviewed in [6, 7]). Emil Fischer had by that time determined the chemical structure of various purines including uric acid and had shown that the latter was an oxidized form of xanthine and hypoxanthine. It was known that uric acid could be synthesized de novo in the liver of birds (Minkowski) or in mammals from small molecules like ammonia and CO_2. Hepatectomy blocked such uric acid synthesis. Miescher had shown that uric acid was produced by the breakdown of nucleic acids. His demonstrated that renal excretion of uric acid was elevated in some but not all gouty patients and that a gouty paroxysm was preceded by a decrease in urinary uric acid excretion followed by an increase. In addition to the theories of primary focal tissue devitalization, various speculations about the systemic causes of hyperuricemia had been advanced based on the physical chemical data of Leibig and others. Neurogenic theories envisioned foci of production of "seed" crystals from the local catabolism of nucleic acids from dead cells in foci of tissue necrosis caused by disturbances in local innervation or from neurogenically induced decreased renal urate excretion (Cullen, Lathame, Luff, Duckworth), with focal toxicity produced by the formation of sphere urates (Mordhorst).

Sokoloff, reviewing the pathology of gout in 1957, considered the tissue deposition of MSU crystals as analogous to calcium phosphate crystal deposition, i. e., either "metastatic" or "dystrophic" [8]. "Metastatic" crystal formation occurred from supersaturated solutions, in preferred sites to be sure, but in tissues that were otherwise healthy. "Dystrophic" crystal formation occurred from not necessarily supersaturated solutions but in focal areas of devitalized tissue.

Factors Responsible for MSU Crystal Deposition

Table 1 summarizes some factors thought to be implicated in MSU crystal deposition. Temperature effects have already been mentioned. I recently encountered an elderly hyperuricemic man who had been treated for several acute attacks of gout in his feet but who had neither tophi or typical radiographic changes. He subsequently developed severe chronic congestive heart failure with an extremely low cardiac output. Multiple small tophi in the skin over all four of his ice-cold extremities formed within a few months with nearly continuous inflammation in the joints of his feet. Thermodynamic data and clinical observations of the centrifugal distribution of the affected tissues support an important role for decreased temperature.

pH was once thought to be important as *uric acid* solubility rises sharply with increasing alkalinity. However, *sodium urate* solubility actually rises as pH falls from 7.4 to 7.0, and the solubility curves of the two substances in buffers [9] or in urine [10] cross one another.

Local tissue edema due to dependency of the lower extremity followed by interstitial fluid resorption at night during recumbency was postulated by Simkin to cause local intrasynovial urate concentrations [11]. This notion was based on his finding that radiolabelled urate cleared from dependent tissue spaces at a rate only half that of tritiated water. This idea could account for the onset of gout at night and its proclivity to attack joints in the foot. It can also account for the occasional patient with crystal-proven gout but without hyperuricemia. Attacks in these individuals are invariably in joints in the foot. This mechanism cannot explain why some individuals and not others develop MSU crystal deposits. Scudamore may have anticipated this idea as he thought congestion of the inferior vena cava somehow was responsible for provoking acute gouty attacks [12].

Urate crystal deposition occurs preferentially in relatively avascular tissue such as bone and dense collagenous structures like tendons, ligaments, joint capsules, and, of course, the avascular articular cartilage. Cartilage absorbs urate, and crystals form readily when cartilage is exposed to saturated solutions of sodium urate in vitro [13, 14]. How do MSU crystals then form in vascularized tissues like skin and synovium? Arthroscopists state that the synovium is often involved before cartilage.

Table 1. Factors of possible importance in monosodium urate crystal deposition

Factor	Estimated relative importance (0 to 4+)	Comment
Temperature	++++	Fits thermodynamic data and clinical observations [3]
pH	±	Important only in uric acid vis-à-vis MSU crystal deposition [9, 10]
Local edema	++	Urate clearance retarded vis-à-vis water; local urate ↑ during fluid reabsorption in recumbent position [11]
Focal necrosis	+	Seems dependent on type of necrosis [7]
Glycosaminoglycan	?	Postulated excluded volume or cation exchange effects [15]
Proteoglycan aggregates	?	Transient increased urate solubility [19, 20]
Rising serum urate	+	Mechanism unclear; increased local solubility if level falls below saturation may cause "shedding" [21, 22]
Falling serum urate	++++	
Relative avascularity	++++	Cartilage nucleates crystals in vitro from supersaturated urate solution [13, 14]
Nucleating factors		
Synovial fluid	?	Gouty fluid much more effective [24]
Lead urate	?	Lead urate very insoluble; nucleates sodium urate [28]
Albumin	?	Epitaxial fit in MSU crystal [16]
"Matrix"	++	Organic material within and between crystals – protein, fat, and carbohydrate [8, 31]
Calcium phosphate	++	Caner–Decker syndrome
Microbiologic products, e.g., fungal	?	Seems far-fetched [30]
Trauma, aging, osteoarthritis	++	Could explain focal deposition of crystals [26]
Macrophage "organelle" sphere	++++	Novel concept based on careful observations [33]

The presence in relatively avascular tissues of glycosaminoglycans which could act as cation exchangers and of proteoglycans or proteoglycan aggregates which might influence urate solubility has led to various proposed pathogenetic mechanisms. Conversely, urate binding to proteins has been invoked as favoring or inhibiting crystal formation. Laurent showed that chondroitin sulfate decreased urate solubility at pH 7.4, which he attributed to an "excluded volume" effect [15]. This would be important only if the small molecule is extensively bound to protein. Many studies have purportedly demonstrated weak binding of a minor portion of urate to various serum proteins (summarized in [16]). While such binding may be important in maintaining urate supersaturation, it is insufficient to produce a significant excluded volume effect in the presence of proteoglycan aggregates. Serum protein binding was postulated to influence renal excretion, especially since some uricosuric drugs displaced urate from its binding site [17], but it is unlikely that protein binding has any such influence because dyes which are known to bind to proteins with much greater avidity are stripped off during glomerular filtration. Sorensen showed definite protein binding by urate at 4°C, less at 30°C, and none at 37°C using equilibrium dialysis [18].

Katz and Schubert reported increased urate solubility with proteoglycan fractions from cartilage [19] later shown to be composed of aggregates [20]. They added protease or hyaluronidase to their solutions, and crystallization of MSU followed. An increased turnover of connective tissue proteoglycans due to similar enzymatic action in vivo was postulated to account for a sudden, focal, decreased urate solubility in proteoglycan-rich tissues such as cartilage, skin, and renal medulla. Perricone and Brandt attributed the results of Katz and Schubert to their use of potassium proteoglycan which caused an apparent increase in urate solubility as the potassium salt is more soluble [20].

Fluctuations in serum urate induced by feasting and alcohol in volunteer gouty subjects were found to induce acute gouty attacks [21]. Such systemic changes were thought to alter the steady state equilibrium between MSU crystals and sodium and urate ions in solution. Attacks of gouty inflammation correlated best with a falling urate level [23]. Acute gouty attacks were often precipitated when allopurinol was first used before it was realized that an antiinflammatory drug should be given routinely to prevent them. If urate levels fall below saturation, crystals slightly could dissolve and, loosened from the organic mold that binds them, shed into the highly vascularized synovial space. This "shedding" phenomenon was postulated to account for acute pseudogout attacks which predictably followed irrigation of joints in patients with calcium pyrophosphate (CPPD) crystal deposition with 40 mM magnesium chloride, a CPPD crystal solubilizer [23]. How a falling urate level which remains supersaturated triggers acute attacks of gout remains unclear but could relate to rapid MSU crystal formation in joint tissues contiguous with the synovial fluid or in the fluid itself.

Histochemical stains have shown lipid in the center of many, but not all, gouty tophi [8]. Cholesterol crystals may be prominent also. Proteinaceous and carbohydrate moieties are seen on occasion [8]. I have found hyaluronidase useful in breaking up tophi into crystal suspensions. These nonurate "matrix" components of tophi have raised much controversy throughout the years with regard to their role in MSU crystal nucleation and growth. Synovial fluid from patients with gout, centrifuged to remove crystals, was much more effective in nucleating MSU crystals than fluids from patients with osteoarthritis [24]. Whether or not ultramicroscopic crystal seeds (colloidal urates) had escaped removal by centrifugation remains unclear. Such crystals have been found (rarely) in gouty synovial fluids as the only species [25]. Increased concentrations of chondroitin sulfate in synovial fluid promoted MSU crystal formation in vitro; trauma, aging, or preexisting joint disease were postulated as producing connective tissue changes favoring MSU crystal deposition [26]. The common occurrence of MSU in Heberden's nodes might be due in part to such changes [27]. Calcium phosphate may have been responsible for nucleation of MSU crystals in the Caner–Decker syndrome of acute periarthritis in hemodialysis patients [27a].

Lead urate is both very insoluble and an excellent nucleating agent for MSU crystals [28]. Subclinical lead toxicity might indeed be very common. If this were a major factor, however, an epidemic of gout in New York City traffic policemen could be expected!

Mycotoxins are known to induce gout in chickens and other avians, probably because of hyperuricemia secondary to renal toxicity [29]. Extrapolations to human gout seem exceedingly farfetched [30].

The matrix of urinary uric acid crystals has attracted a lot of attention. Heparan sulfate, albumin, and Tamm–Horsfall mucoprotein are major components [31]. Serum albumin can be incorporated by epitaxial overgrowth in MSU crystals grown in vitro [16]. An analysis of natural MSU crystals for intra- as opposed to intercrystalline matrix components has not yet been accomplished. Certainly, many molecules adsorb to urate crystal surfaces (summarized in [32]). Whether any of these have a bearing on crystal formation is unclear.

A careful histologic study of excised gouty olecranon bursae revealed small, spherical arrays of multinucleated giant cells and macrophages enclosing a necrotic tissue matrix devoid of MSU crystals [33]. The necrotic center often contained cell membranes (lipids) identified by monoclonal antibodies as belonging to the same lineage as the cells arranged in the spheres. Somewhat larger, and presumably more mature, tophi held MSU crystals. Still larger crystal masses were achieved by fusion of the smaller masses. History has repeated itself with Epstein's theory rising again with modern scientific support! The authors postulated that the spheres of macrophages and giant cells derived from macrophages form a secretory organ concentrating urates inside the sphere by active anion transport, a phenomenon just recently described for macrophages [34]. MSU crystals eventually nucleate and grow inside the sphere to initiate the tophus. This theory has several attractive features. It creates an avascular environment even in highly vascularized tissues. The sphere formation of cells is nearly universally observed around small tophi. It potentially could explain why only some hyperuricemic subjects deposit crystals. The etiology of the cellular sphere and the nature of its necrotic central focus remain a mystery (? Colloidal sphere urates). Such cells obviously cannot explain MSU crystal deposits in cartilage.

References

1. McCarty DJ (1985) Pathogenesis and treatment of crystal-induced inflammation. In: McCarty DJ (ed) Arthritis and Allied Conditions, 10th Ed., Lea & Febiger, Philadelphia
2. Holmes EW (1985) Clinical Gout and the pathogenesis of hyperuricemia. In: McCarty DJ (ed). Arthritis and Allied Conditions, 10th Ed, Lea & Febiger, Philadelphia
3. Loeb JN (1972) The influence of temperature on the solubility of monosodium urate. Arthritis Rheum 15: 189–192
4. Garrod AB (1876) A treatise on Gout and Rheumatic Gout (Rheumatoid Arthritis). 3rd Ed, London, Longemans, Green
5. Riehl G (1897) Zur Anatomie der Gicht. Wien Klin Wochenschr 10: 761
6. Freudweiler M (1964) Studies on the nature of gouty tophi, an abridged translation with comments. Brill JM, McCarty DJ. Ann Intern Med 60: 486–505 [Original Deutsch Arch für Klin Med 63: 266, 1899]
7. Freudweiler M (1965) Experimental investigations into the origin of gouty tophi. Translated by Brill JM, McCarty DJ, Arthritis Rheum 8: 267–288 [Original Deutsch Arch für Klin Med 69: 155, 1901]
8. Sokoloff L (1957) The pathology of gout. Metabolism 6: 230–243
9. Wilcox WR, Khalaf A, Weinberger A, Kippen I, Klinenberg JR (1972) Solubility of uric acid and monosodium urate. Med & Biol Eng 10: 522–531
10. Shimizu T, Nishikawa M, Matsushige H (1989) The solubility of uric acid and monosodium urate in urine. Adv Exp Med Biol 253A: 215–218
11. Simkin P (1977) The pathogenesis of podagra. Ann Intern Med 86: 230–233
12. Scudamore C (1819) A treatise on the nature and cure of gout and rheumatism. 1st American edition, Edward Earle, Philadelphia, p 182
13. Brugsch T, Citron J (1908) Ueber die Absorption der Harnsäure durch Knorpel. Ztschr f exp Path v Therap 5: 401–405
14. Roberts W (1892) The Croonian lectures on the chemistry and therapeutics of uric acid gravel and gout. Brit M J 2: 61–65
15. Laurent TC (1964) Solubility of sodium urate in the presence of chondroitin-4-sulphate. Nature 202: 1334
16. Perl-Treves D, Addadi L (1988) A structural approach to pathological crystallizations: Gout: the possible role of albumin in sodium urate crystallization. Proc R Soc Lond [B] 235: 145–159
17. Kippen I, Klinenberg JR, Weinberger A, Wilcox WR (1974) Factors affecting urate solubility in vitro. Ann Rheum Dis 33: 313–317
18. Sorensen LB, Personal communication.
19. Katz WA, Schubert M (1970) The interaction of monosodium urate with connective tissue components. J Clin Invest 49: 1783–1789

20. Perricone E, Brandt K (1978) Enhancement of urate solubility by connective tissue. Arthritis Rheum 21: 453–460
21. Maclachlan MJ, Rodnan GP (1967) Effects of food, fast and alcohol on serum uric acid and acute attacks of gout. Am J Med 42: 38–57
22. Rodnan GP (1980) The pathogenesis of aldermanic gout: procatarctic role of fluctuation in serum urate concentrations in gouty arthritis provoked by feast and alcohol. Arthritis Rheum 23: 737
23. Bennett RM, Lehr JR, McCarty DJ (1976) Crystal shedding and acute pseudo-gout: an hypothesis based on a therapeutic failure. Arthritis Rheum 19: 93–97
24. Tak HK, Cooper SM, Wilcox WR (1980) Studies on the nucleation of mono-sodium urate at 37°C. Arthritis Rheum 23: 574–580
25. Honig S, Gorevic P, Hoffstein S, Weissmann G (1979) Crystal deposition disease. Diagnosis by electron microscopy. Am J Med 63: 161–164
26. Burt HM, Dutt YC (1986) Growth of monosodium urate monohydrate crystals: effect of cartilage and synovial fluid components on in vitro growth rates. Ann Rheum Dis 45: 858–864
27. Lally EV, Zimmerman B, Ho G, Kaplan SR (1989) Urate-mediated inflammation in nodal osteoarthritis: clinical and roengenographic correlations. Arthritis Rheum 32: 86–90
27a. Caner SEZ, Decker JH
28. Tak HK, Wilcox WR, Cooper SM (1981) The effect of lead upon urate nucleation. Arthritis Rheum 24: 1291–1296
29. Pegram RA, Wyatt RD (1981) Avian gout caused by oosporein, a mycotoxin produced by chaetomium trilaterale. Poultry Sci 60: 2429–2440
30. Costantini AV (1989) Fungalbionics: a new concept of the etiology of gout, hyperuricemia and their related diseases. Adv Exp Med Biol 253A: 261–268
31. Iwata H, Kamei B, Abe Y, Nishio S, Wakatsuki A, Ochi K, Takeuchi M (1988) The organic matrix of urinary uric acid crystals. J Urol 139: 607–610
32. Terkeltaub RA, Ginsberg MH, McCarty DJ (1989) Pathogenesis and treatment of crystalinduced inflammation. In: McCarty DJ (ed.) Arthritis and Allied Conditions, 11th ed. Lea & Febiger, Philadelphia
33. Palmer DG, Highton J, Hessian PA (1989) Development of the gout tophus: an hypothesis. Am J Clin Path 91: 190–195
34. Steinberg TH, Newman AS, Swanson JA, Silverstein SC (1987) Macrophages possess probenecid-inhibitable organic anion transporters that remove fluorescent dyes from the cytoplasmic matrix. J Cell Biol 105: 2695–2702.

J. G. PUIG

In certain clinical situations, serum urate levels become very high but we do not see the clinical consequences of possible urate precipitation. We believe that in these cases urate does not precipitate, even if serum urate rises above 15 to 20 mg/dl (above 900 µmol/l). A good example would be subjects with tuberculosis, especially common in AIDS patients and who are treated with with pyrazinamide. Serum urate levels in these patients increase to above 10 mg/dl (above 600 µmol/l) but they do not exhibit clinical manifestations.

B. EMMERSON

I would like to make a comment about the time factor and hyperuricaemia in HPRT deficiency. Many of these patients have normal serum urate concentrations for many years while they are able to excrete the excessive amounts of urate produced. They become hyperuricaemic only when excretion cannot keep up with production, so that they may be quite old before they develop hyperuricaemia.

However, I have understood this to mean that there is probably much more asymptomatic urate crystal deposition in tissues than is apparent from reliance on symptoms in the joints of hyperuricaemic patients.

K. L. SCHMIDT

We have heard from Dr. Scott that urate tophi never can be observed in muscle. However, in severe cases of CPPD-deposition disease we can see calcifications in the adductor muscles of the legs. What is the biochemical reason for this discrepancy between the behaviour of urate and CPPD crystals?

3

Urate Depositions in Tissues

W. Mohr

In histological tissue sections, monosodium urate crystals appear as collections of negative birefringent, needle-like deposits (Fig. 1 a, b). Their electron microscopic equivalent is crystals with a focal parallel arrangement of their long axes (Fig. 1 c, d). Vacuoles inside the crystals are due to the effect of the electron beam (Pritzker et al. 1978). However, the finding of these crystals in histological sections is dependent on several conditions that will be briefly discussed at the end of this chapter.

An increased serum uric acid content will affect the kidney (Fig. 2). The acute increased excretion of uric acid, occurring in situations of an augmented cell turnover as in the neonatal period or with some haematological malignancies, may be followed by acute uric acid nephropathy ("uric infarction" in the German literature). The macroscopic appearance has been described by Garrod (1859) as "streaks of white matter seen at the apex of each pyramid, and running up in the direction of the tubuli" (Fig. 3 a). Histologically, the crystals are preferentially located in the urinary collecting tubules. In most instances these crystalline accumulations are surrounded by an intact epithelial layer – if epithelial cells become necrotic (Fig. 3 b), crystals may penetrate the basement membrane and eventually appear in the renal interstitial tissue. A similar mechanism may be at work in the pathogenesis of chronic urate nephropathy (Fig. 3 c). According to the results of Farebrother et al. (1975) it is assumed that intratubular crystals destroy the epithelial cells and basement membranes and then gain access to the interstitial tissue of the kidney. In this location they evoke a foreign body reaction characterised by foci of multinuclear giant cells (Fig. 3 d). Interstitial medullary microtophi of this kind were observed in the kidneys of 8% of unselected autopsies in Brisbane (Linnane et al. 1981). An accompanying "unspecific" chronic inflammation may lead to morphological changes that are similar to those of interstitial nephritis (Fig. 3 c).

An increased serum uric acid content must be in equilibrium with that of the interstitial fluid. This situation is reflected by investigations of the periarticular adipose tissue in cases of gout. "Thick frozen sections" of alcohol-dehydrated adipose tissue reveal collections of crystals often imitating the outlines of the adipocytes (Fig. 4 a–c). The raised level of uric acid in the interstitial tissue also implicates an increased concentration in the synovial fluid (Fig. 2). From this situation it may be concluded that the tissues of the

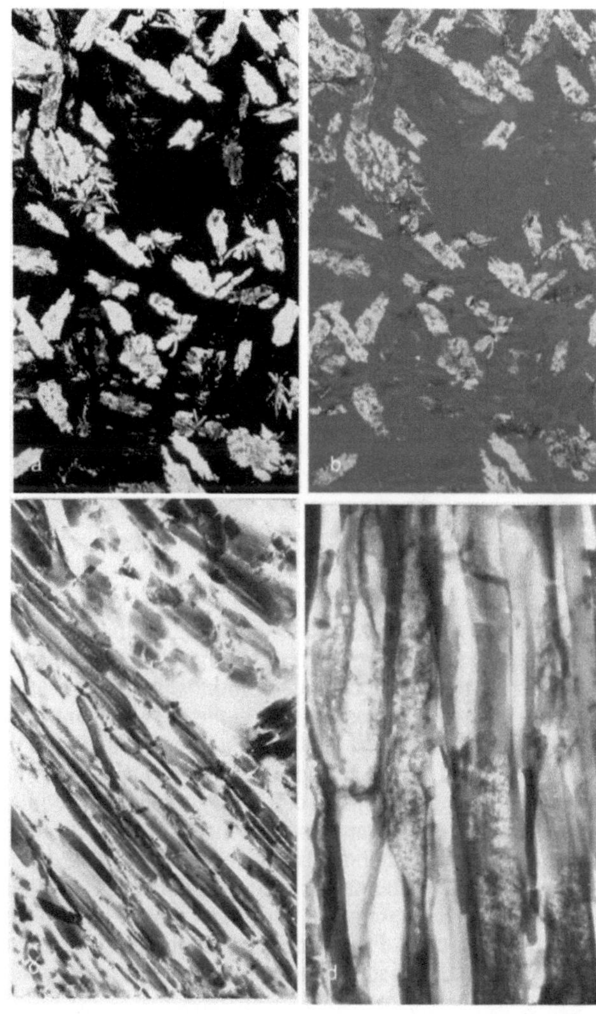

Fig. 1 a – d. Structure of monosodium urate crystals in tissue sections. **a** Urate crystals under conventional light microscopy. H&E, ×85. **b** Identical area of the crystals under compensated light microscopy. ×85. **c** Urate crystals under transmission electron microscopy. ×5700. **d** Urate crystals under transmission electron microscopy with demonstration of internal vacuolisation. ×22 000

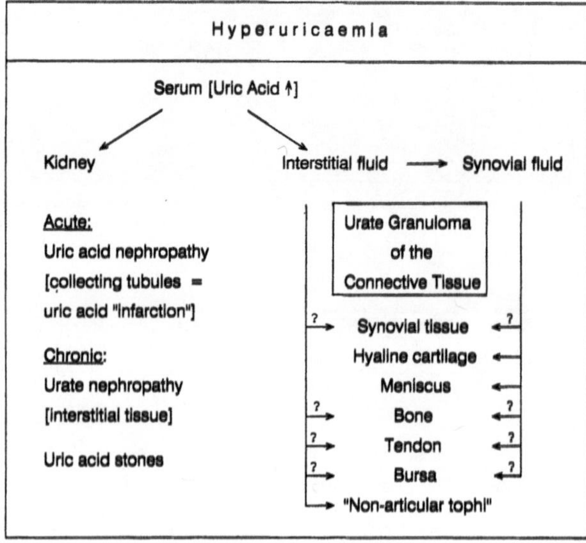

Fig. 2. Hyperuricaemia and the possible consequences in the kidney and the connective tissue

locomotory system may be affected in two ways. Except for hyaline cartilage, menisci and places in which non-articular tophi (Table 1) develop, the way by which the tissues become affected is not well documented (Fig. 2).

For the pathologist, crystals of monosodium urate are only one side of the story – the more important side is the development of reactions against the local accumulation of crystals. Crystalline deposits and the subsequent cellular events lead to the formation of the urate granuloma of the connective tissue – these granulomata can be regarded as the equivalent of the tophus, representing an "inflammation-induced nodule" (Zetkin et al. 1964). The urate granuloma may be defined as "circumscribed deposits of sodium urate in an usually acellular matrix surrounded by cells" that belong to the mononuclear phagocytic system and which can fuse to multinuclear giant cells of the foreign body type. From immunohistological investigations, Palmer et al. (1987) concluded that the cellular components of the gouty tophus have a low

Table 1. Localisation of non-articular tophi

Ear
Eye (Zoller et al. 1985; Martinez-Cordero et al. 1986)
Vocal cord (Virchow 1868)
Mitral valve (Bunim and McEwen 1940; Traut et al. 1954)
Intervertebral disc (Das De 1988)
Dermis (Niemi 1977)
Cushing striae (Palacios-Boix et al. 1984)

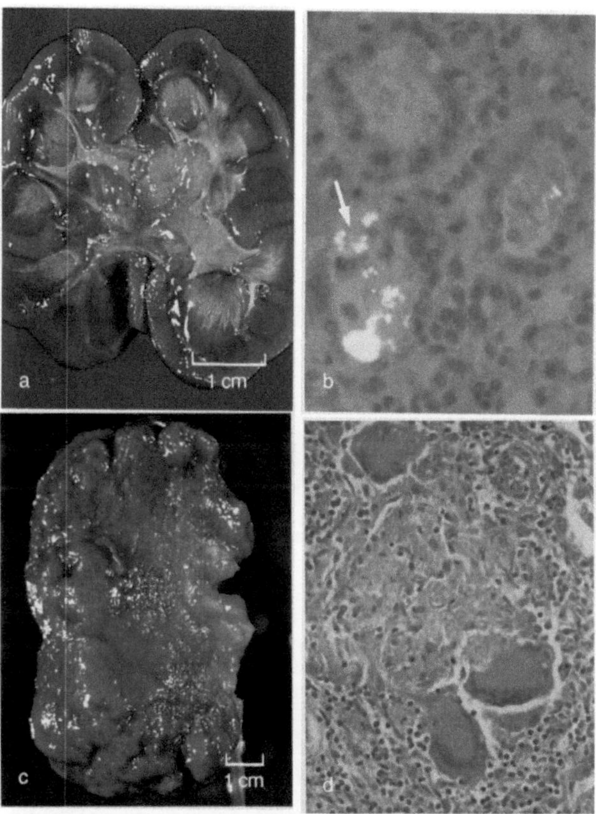

Fig. 3 a – d. Kidney in hyperuricaemia. **a** Uric acid nephropathy with accumulation of uric acid crystals in the collecting tubuli of the pyramids. **b** Histological equivalent: urate crystals inside the tubuli with focal loss of epithelial cells (*arrow*). H&E (polarized light), × 330. **c, d** Chronic urate nephropathy. **c** Macroscopical appearance: advanced interstitial nephritis. **d** Foreign body granuloma in the interstitial tissue of this kidney. H&E, × 220

turnover in contrast to the cells of the rheumatoid nodule, indicating that there is only a low chemotactic activity in the urate granuloma.

If the crystals of the granuloma are partially or totally dissolved, the structure of the matrix becomes apparant. In most instances, it consists of a fine, fibrillar, acellular area that is more or less sharply demarcated from the surrounding cellular infiltrate (Fig. 4 d). If the collagenous fibrils are stained, it becomes obvious that inside these acellular areas with remnants of urate crystals, collagenous fibrils are absent – however, the isolated granuloma may be surrounded by bundles of collagen (Fig. 4 e).

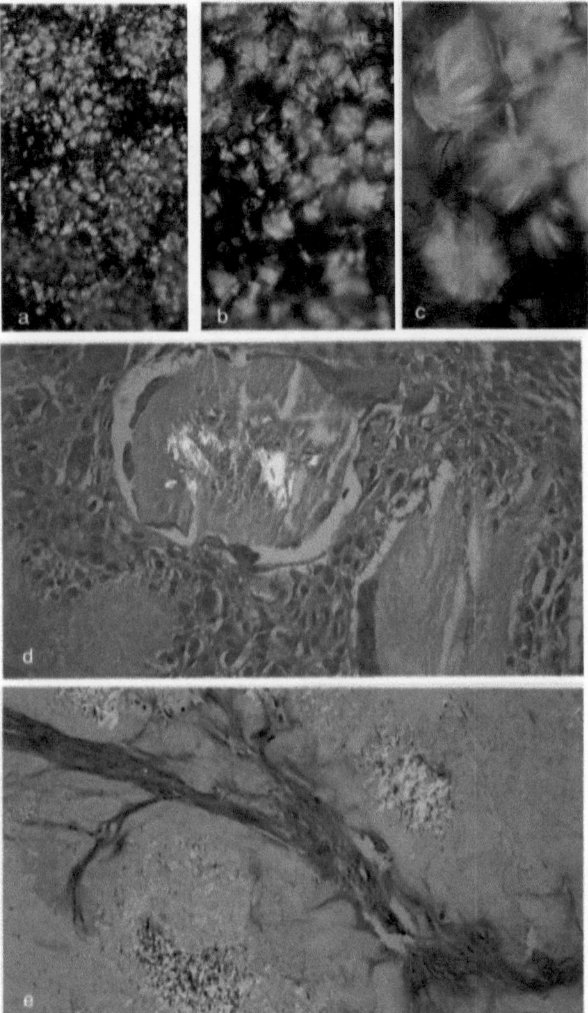

Fig. 4. a – c "Thick frozen section" of the periarticular adipose tissue in a case of gouty arthropathy: crystals imitating the structure of adipocytes. Unstained section, **a** ×35, **b** ×85, **c** ×220 (polarized light). **d** Urate granulomata with remnants of urate crystals in an acellular matrix surrounded by mononuclear phagocytes and multinuclear giant cells. H&E (polarized light), ×220. **e** Urate granulomata separated by collagenous fibres. Azan (polarized light), ×85

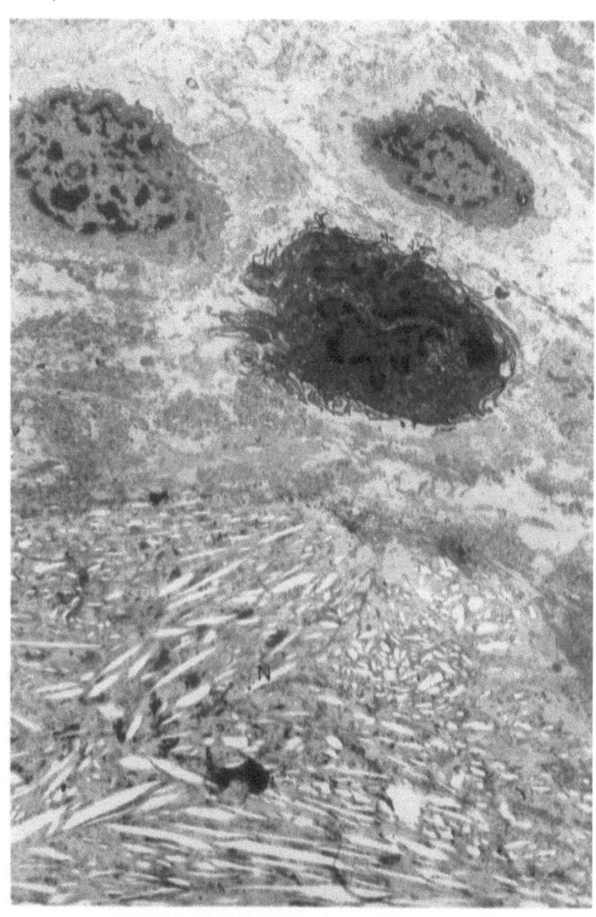

Fig. 5. Electron microscopy study of a urate granuloma. Necrotic area (*N*) with clefts of dissolved urate crystals is surrounded by cells of the mononuclear phagocytic system. × 4600

Electron microscopy study demonstrates the necrotic zone with clefts of dissolved urate crystals and a surrounding of cells with many irregular microvilli (Fig. 5). The ultrastructure of the matrix may indicate the age of these granulomata. Younger ones consist of clefts of dissolved urate crystals with collagenous fibrils and remnants of destroyed cells (Fig. 6). Older granulomata are composed preferentially of an amorphous or fine granular matrix, without collagenous fibrils (Gieseking 1972) or cellular remnants, intermingled with clefts of the dissolved urate crystals (Fig. 7). The question of by which way these granulomata develop is not clearly answered. In a recent

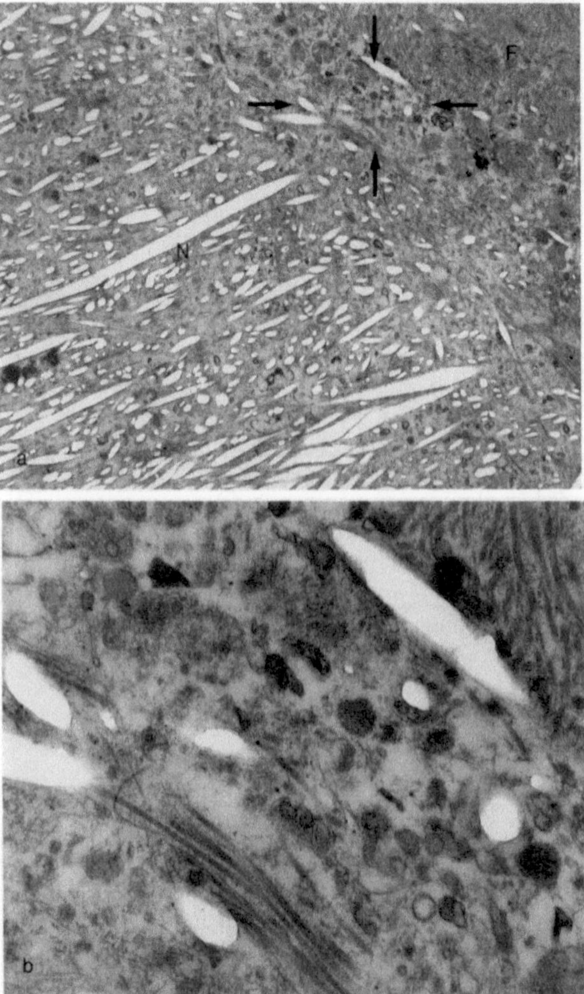

Fig. 6 a, b. Electron microscopy study of a urate granuloma. **a** Central necrotic area (*N*) with clefts of dissolved urate crystals surrounded by a matrix of collagenous fibrils (*F*). ×5700. **b** Higher magnification of the area demarcated with *arrows* in **a**: between the clefts of the dissolved urate crystals lie remnants of collagenous fibrils and necrotic cells. ×27 500

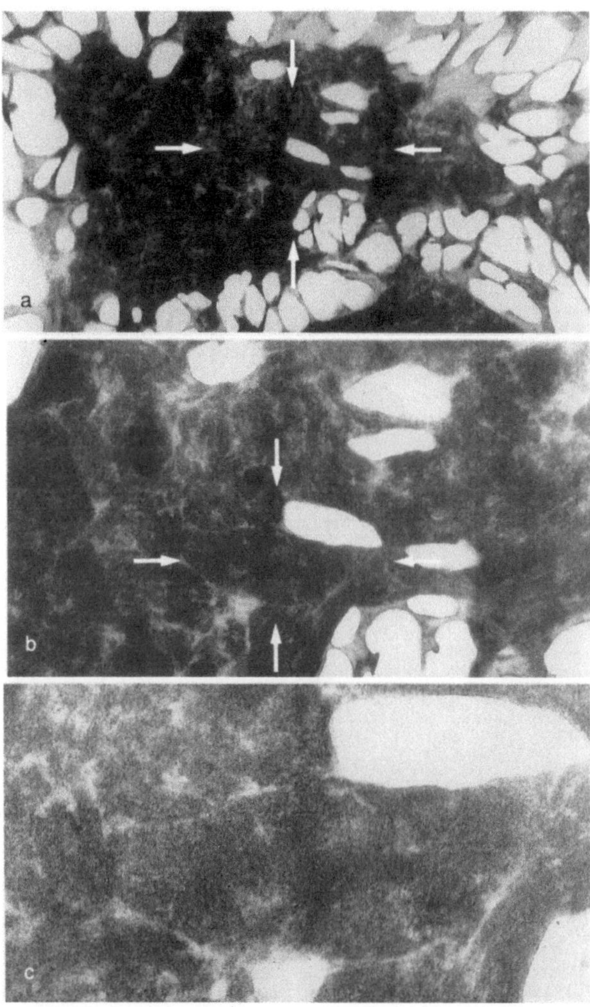

Fig. 7a–c. Electron microscopy study of the central area of an urate granuloma consisting of a fine fibrillar material with clefts of the dissolved urate crystals. **a** ×17600. **b** Higher magnification of the area demarcated with *arrows* in **a**. ×35000. **c** Higher magnification of the area demarcated with *arrows* in **b**. ×89000

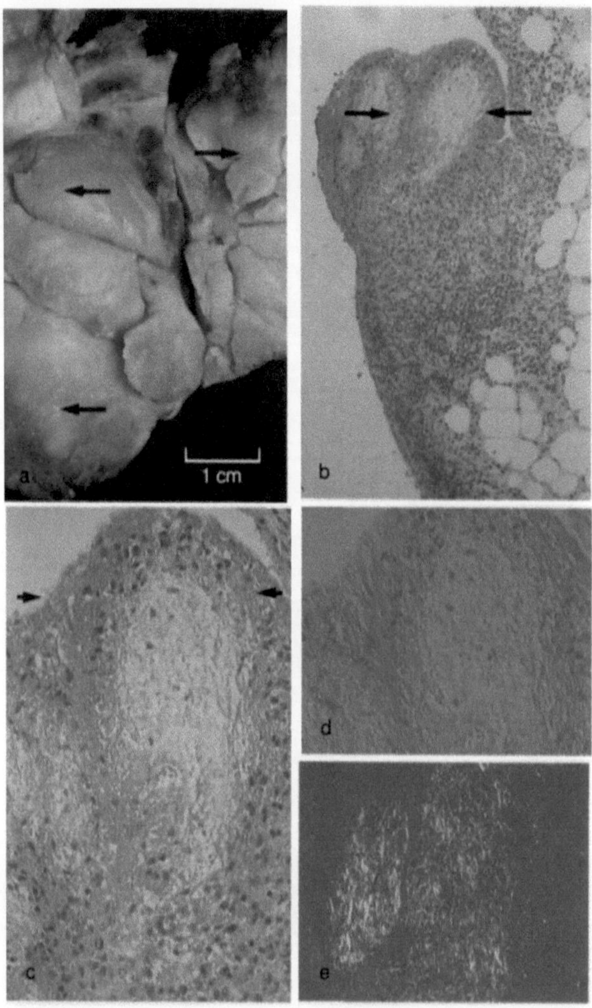

Fig. 8a–e. Synovial tissue of a patient with recent onset of gouty arthritis (alcohol-dehydrated tissue) **a** Macroscopic view of the synovial adipose tissue with small white urate spots (*arrows*). **b** Urate granuloma (*arrows*) in the superficial area of the adipose synovial tissue. H&E, ×85. **c** Higher magnification of the area marked with *arrows* in **b**: loose network of fibrillar material surrounded by mononuclear cells and covered by fibrin. H&E, ×220. **d** In the polarized light a conventionally stained section does not contain crystalline deposits (from area demarked with *arrows* in **c**). H&E, ×220. **e** In a subsequent unstained section of the same area a loose network of urate crystals is seen under polarized light. ×220

paper by Palmer et al. (1989), it is assumed that "acini" of macrophages develop about an acellular or necrotic center and transport urate from the interstitial fluid into this central zone.

Gout preferentially affects the organs or the locomotory system. However, with regard to the joints it is unknown in which place urate crystals primarily appear. According to Brogsitter (1926), the cartilage is primarily affected; Uehlinger (1976) assumed that the first crystals develop in the synovial fluid, and Sokoloff (1957) as well as Agudelo and Schumacher (1973) favour the synovial membrane as the place of the initial crystallisation. Nevertheless, the morphological changes that appear in the different structures of the loco-motory system are well-known.

The *synovial tissue* may exhibit several morphological changes. In the early stages of the disease the adipose synovial tissue is covered with small grey spots (Fig. 8a). Light microscopy shows in this instance in the superficial areas of the adipose synovial tissue acellular zones of a fine fibrillar matrix surrounded by infiltrations of mononuclear cells in a loose arrangement. These areas are covered by a tiny layer of fibrin (Fig. 8b, c). In H&E-stained sections of alcohol-dehydrated tissue the crystals are dissolved (Fig. 8d), but they can be demonstrated inside these acellular zones in un-stained sections, in which the crystals are preserved (Fig. 8e). In more advanced cases a similar macroscopic appearance may be observed – the synovial adipose tissue shows a stippled surface (Fig. 9a). The histological equivalent consists of acellular foci that are surrounded by mononuclear phagocytes and some multinuclear giant cells (Fig. 9b, c). Also in these alcohol-dehydrated specimens crystals are usually dissolved by the conventional H&E staining – however, they are preserved in unstained sections and appear as dense crystalline collections (Fig. 9d). More advanced cases exhibit a thickened synovial membrane (Fig. 10a) with urate granulomata in the superficial synovial areas (Fig. 10b). Outside these granulomata, a dense cellular infiltrate of lymphocytes and plasmolytes is present (Fig. 10c, d). In some cases, a dense fibrinous exudate covers the synovial surface (Fig. 11a) in the region of the granulomatous inflammation (Fig. 11b). Synovial villi contain focal accumulations of lymphocytes and plasmocytes as well as small urate granulomata (Fig. 11c) surrounded by mononuclear cells and some polymorphonuclear granulocytes (Fig. 11d). From these histological appearances it may be assumed that urate preferentially gains access to the synovial tissue via the synovial fluid.

The morphological changes of the *hyaline cartilage* are also well-known. In advanced cases, the surface of the cartilage is covered by urate (Kersley et al. 1950). Histological changes consist of superficial deposits of urate in the cartilaginous matrix (Fig. 12) as described by Garrod (1859) and Brogsitter (1926). The surface of the cartilage often exhibits a fine granular eosinophilic appearance (Fig. 12c, d), indicating that crystals have been dissolved by the staining method from these areas. A cellular pannus tissue may grow over or into the cartilage (Mohr 1984; Fig. 12a). In more advanced cases the cartilage

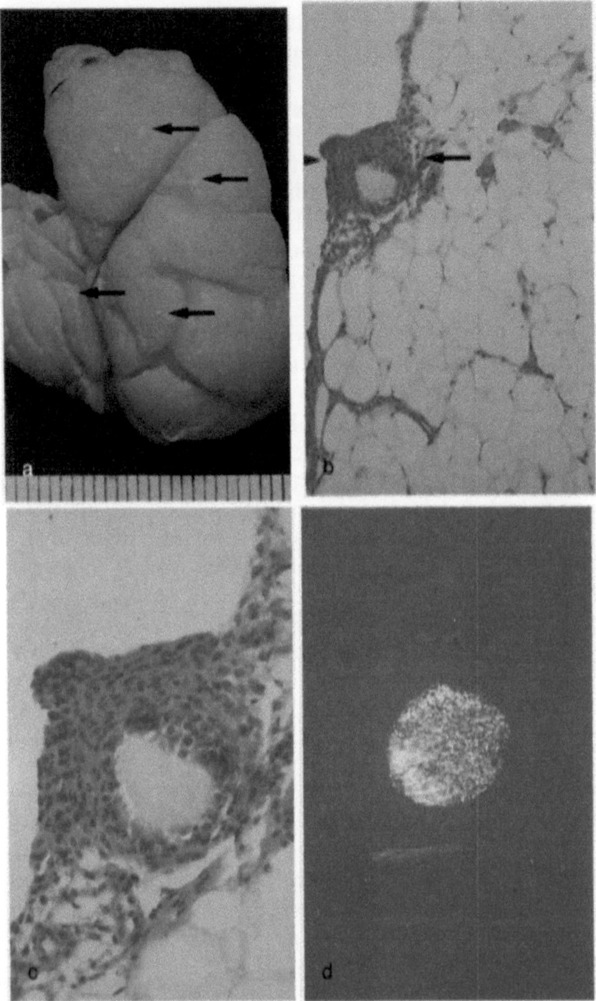

Fig. 9 a – d. Synovial tissue of a patient with recent onset of gouty arthritis (alcohol-dehydrated tissue). **a** Macroscopic view of the adipose synovial tissue covered by small white urate spots (*arrows*). **b** Histological section demonstrating a urate granuloma in the superficial synovial fat pad. H&E, ×85. **c** Higher magnification of the granuloma in **b** (*arrows*): central acellular area surrounded by mononuclear phagocytes and some multinuclear giant cells. H&E, ×220. **d** Under polarized light urate crystals are seen in the unstained section of this granuloma. ×220

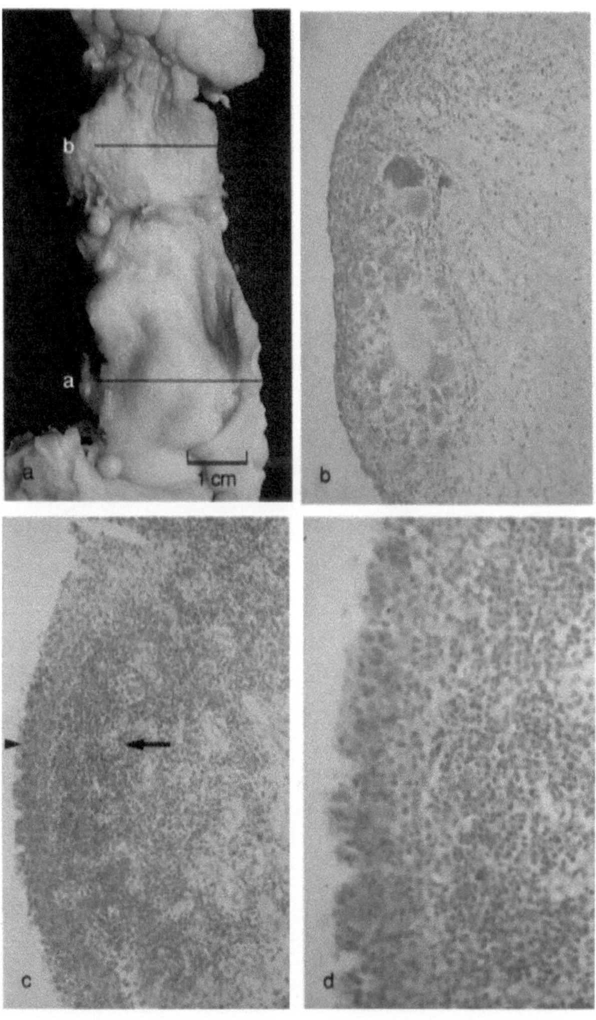

Fig. 10 a–d. Synovial tissue of a patient with longer-standing gouty arthritis (formalin-fixed tissue). **a** Macroscopic view of the synovial tissue with a smooth surface. **b** Urate granuloma in the superficial synovial tissue from *a* in **a**. H&E, ×85. **c** Synovial tissue with a dense chronic inflammatory infiltration (area *b* in **a**). H&E, ×85. **d** Higher magnification of the area marked with *arrows* in **c**: under the broadened synovial cell layer a dense infiltrate of lymphocytes and predominantly plasmocytes. H&E, ×220

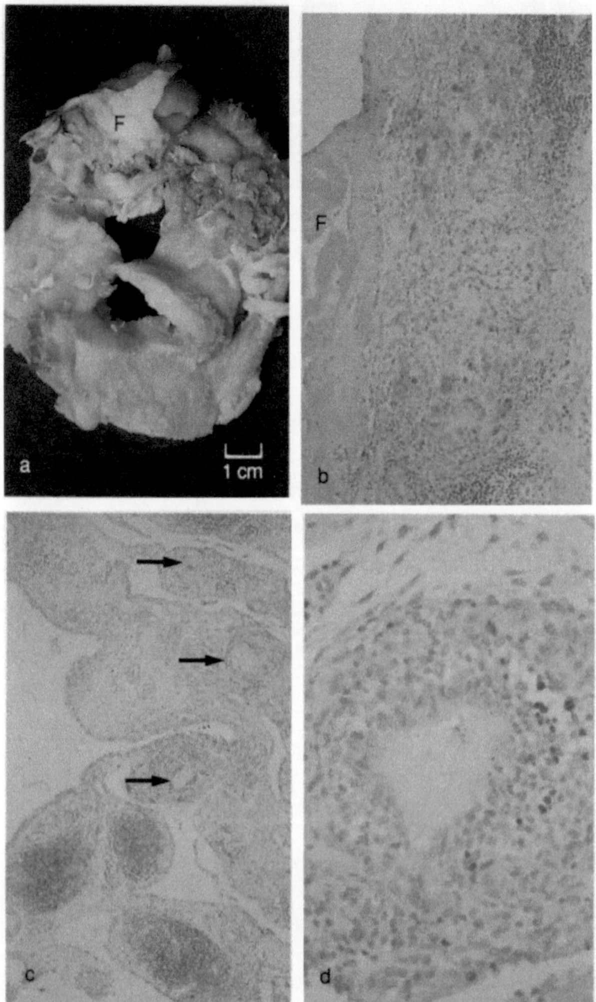

Fig. 11 a–d. Synovial tissue of a patient with longer-standing gouty arthritis (formalin-fixed tissue). **a** Macroscopic view of the synovial tissue focally covered by a dense layer of fibrin (*F*). **b** Under the fibrinous exudate (*F*) granulomata with multinuclear giant cells. H&E, ×85. **c** Synovial villi with a follicular lympho-plasmocytic infiltrate and some urate granulomata (*arrows*). H&E, ×35. **d** Granuloma in a synovial villus consisting of an acellular area surrounded by mononuclear cells and some polymorphonuclear granulocytes. Naphthol-AS-D-chloroacetate esterase, ×220

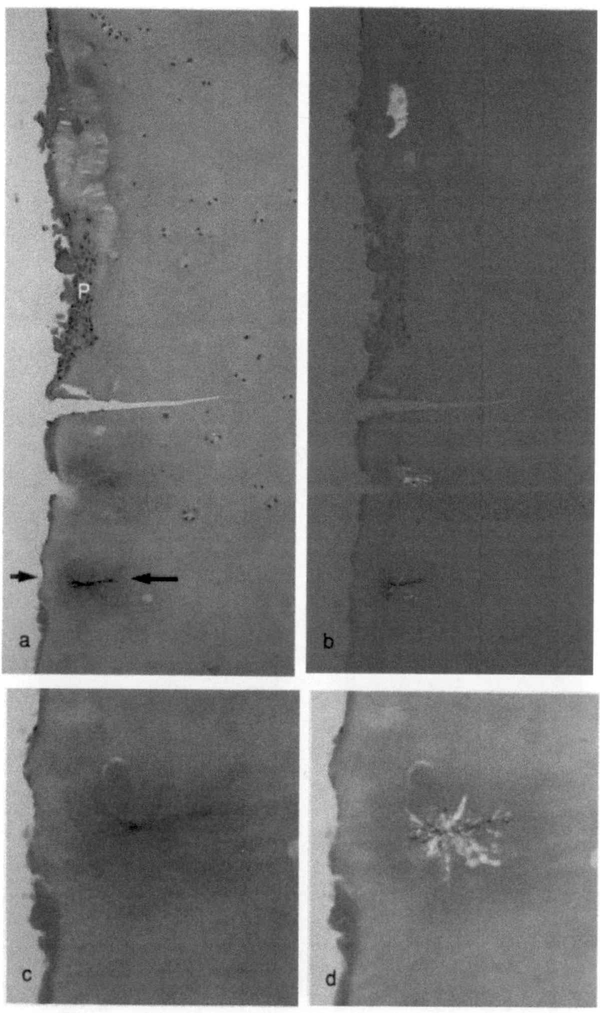

Fig. 12 a – d. Hyaline cartilage of a patient with gouty arthritis. **a, b** Superficial areas of the hyaline cartilage with urate deposits and a cellular pannus tissue (*P*). H&E, (**b** polarized light), ×85. **c, d** Higher magnification of the area demarcated with *arrows* in **a**: focal collections of urate crystals in a cartilaginous matrix without chondrocytes and a fine fibrillated surface with a strong eosinophilie appearance. H&E (**d** polarized light), ×220

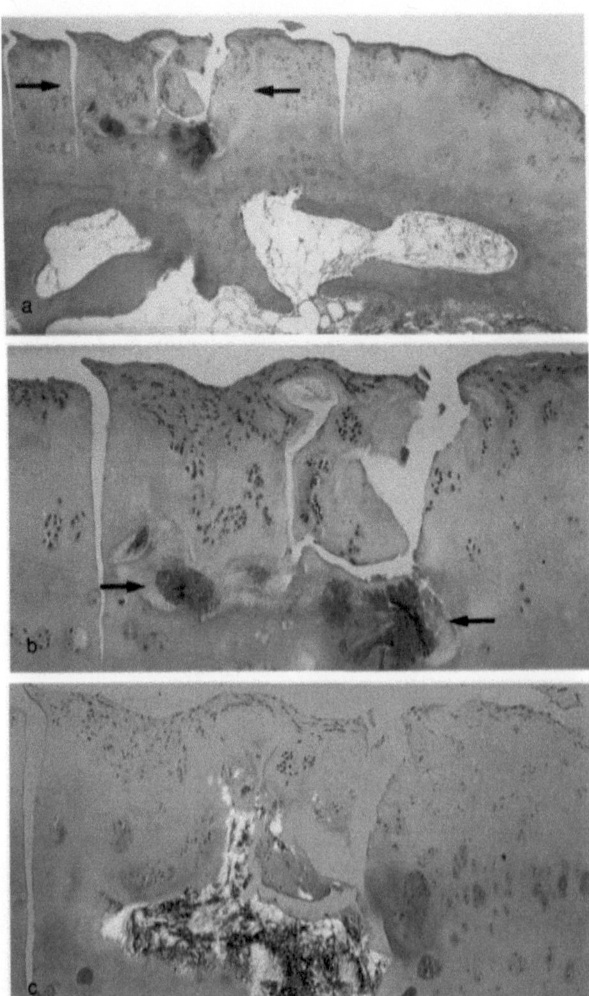

Fig. 13 a–c. Hyaline cartilage of a patient with gouty arthritis. **a** Fibrillated cartilage with focal deposits of urate. H&E, ×35. **b** Higher magnification of the area demarcated with *arrows* in **a**: partially necrotic cartilage with fissures and clusters of chondrocytes and urate crystals (*arrows*). H&E, ×85. **c** Proteoglycan loss of cartilage in the same area. Safranin 0 (polarized light), ×85

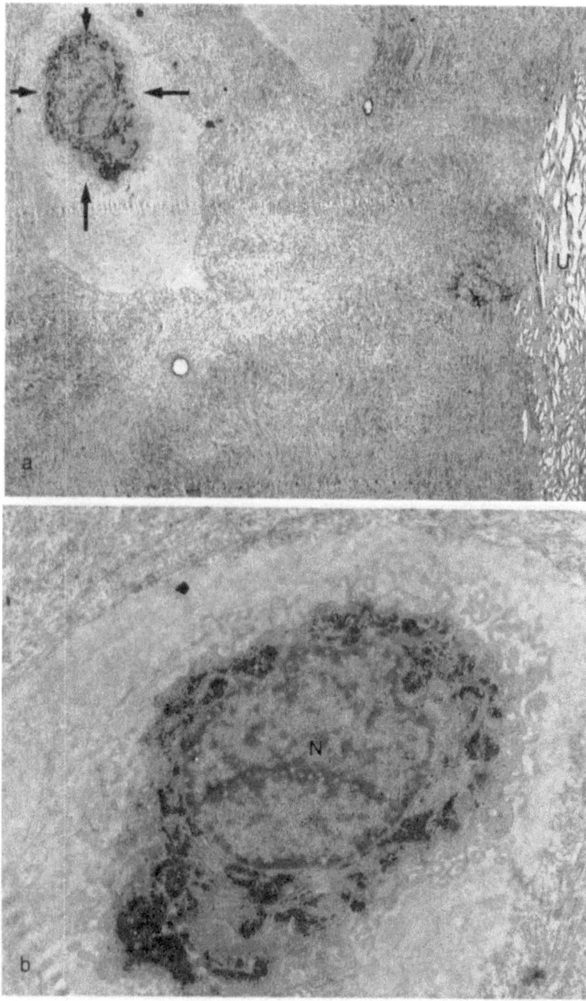

Fig. 14 a, b. Electron microscopic view of the cartilage of a patient with gouty arthritis. **a** Cartilaginous matrix with a chondrocyte in the neighbourhood of a matrix with clefts of the dissolved urate crystals (*U*). ×2200. **b** Higher magnification of the chondrocyte demarcated in **a** with *arrows*. Nucleus (*N*) is well preserved, and cytoplasm is rich in glycogen. ×7300

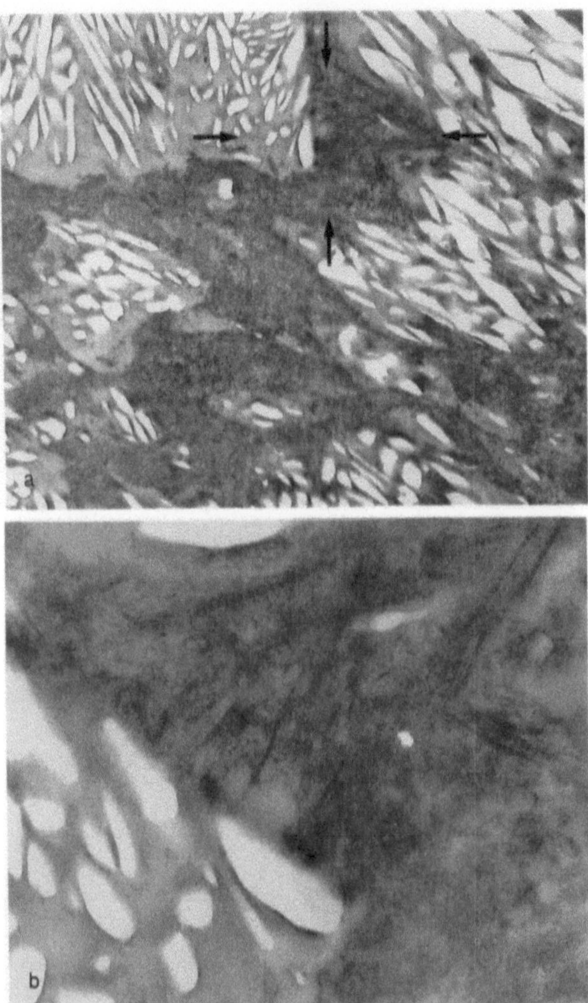

Fig. 15 a, b. Ultrastructural study of the cartilaginous matrix with urate deposits.
a Cartilaginous matrix with clefts of dissolved urate crystals and a fine granular
matrix. ×7300. **b** Higher magnification of the area designated with *arrows* in **a**: the
cartilaginous matrix consists of remnants of collagenous fibrils and a fine granular
material. ×27 500

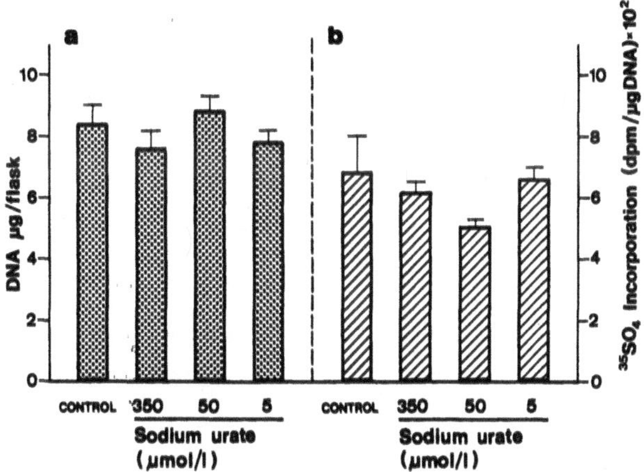

Fig. 16 a, b. Results of the in vitro growth of chondrocytes with sodium urate. **a** DNA content/flask for control and test (sodium urate: 5, 50 and 350 mM) groups. Mean values ± SD of the mean; seven observations per group. No statistically significant differences at the 1% level of significance. **b** Incorporation of $^{35}SO_4$ in cartilage glycosaminoglycans by control and test (sodium urate: 5, 50 and 350 μM) chondrocytes. Mean values ± SD of the mean; seven observations per group. No statistically significant differences at the 1% level of significance. (From Kirkpatrick et al. 1981)

is fissured, and urate deposits are present in the neighbourhood of the clefts (Fig. 13). From safranin-0-stained specimens it becomes evident that there is an advanced depletion of proteoglycans (Fig. 13 c). Near the cartilaginous fissures, areas with a reduced content of chondrocytes as well as clusters of chondrocytes are present (Fig. 13 b). Thus, morphological alterations similar to the osteoarthrotic process characterise this stage of the disease.

Under electron microscopy study a cartilaginous matrix with clefts (Hirohata et al. 1981), indicating dissolved urate crystals, is seen (Fig. 14 a). In the neighbourhood of the urate deposits, chondrocytes rich in glycogen may be present (Fig. 14). The cartilaginous matrix surrounding the clefts consists of fine collagenous fibrils and deposits of a granular material (Fig. 15). From the morphological changes it is apparant that urate reaches the cartilage via the synovial fluid – nevertheless, the mechanism leading to its accumulation inside the cartilaginous matrix is not known.

As light microscopic investigations indicated the occurrence of necrotic chondrocytes, we became interested in the question of whether urate may alter the function of chondrocytes in vitro. From Fig. 16 it can be seen that different concentrations of sodium urate affect neither the proliferation of chondrocytes nor their ability to synthesize glycosaminoglycans. It can be deduced that urate has no deleterious effect on the tested functions of these cells.

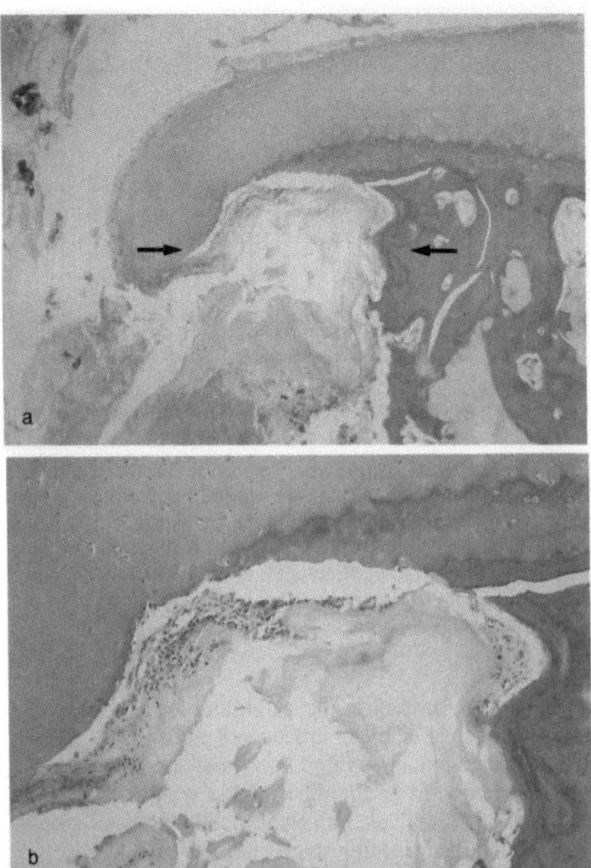

Fig. 17 a, b. Paraosseous tophus invading the subcartilaginous bone. **a** Tophus has replaced the paraosseous bone. H&E, × 35. **b** Higher magnification of the area designated with *arrows* in **a**: acellular tophus under the hyaline cartilage with a cellular reaction in the periphery. H&E, × 85

Synovial fluid urate may also reach the *menisci*, leading to huge urate deposits inside the meniscal substance with subsequent destruction.

Bones may become involved primarily through intraosseous tophi or secondarily through the synovial fluid in patients with cartilage and bone defects or through the invasion of periosteal tophi. From morphological observations it seems reasonable to assume that the two latter mechanisms are the main events leading to bone destruction. In particular, periarticular tophi may

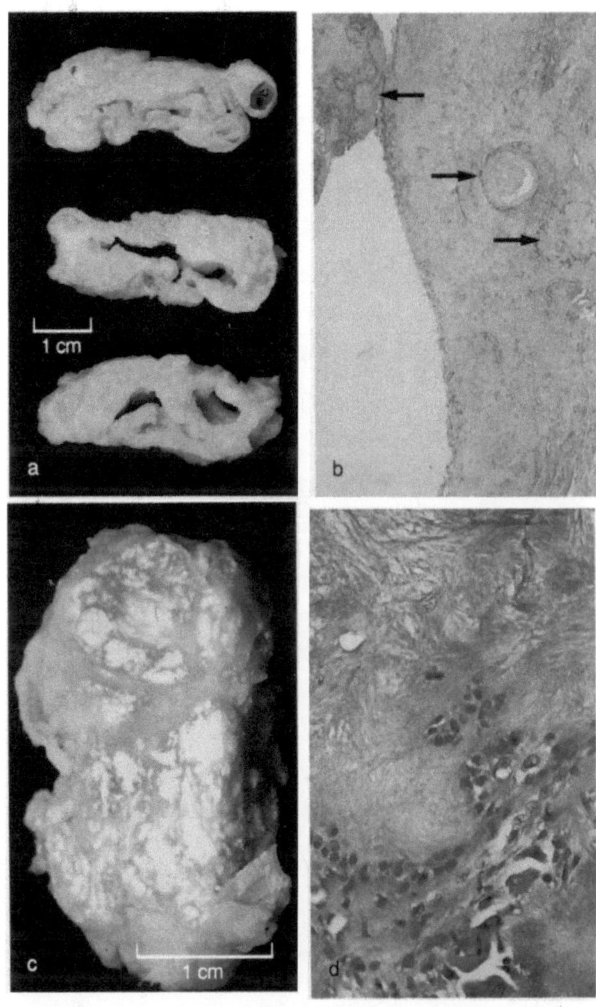

Fig. 18 a–d. Bursal involvement in a patient with gouty arthritis. **a** Macroscopic view of the wall of a bursa with a central lumen. **b** In this bursal wall are urate granulomata (*arrows*). H&E, ×15. **c** Macroscopically, the bursa consists of fibrous tissue with urate deposits. **d** Acellular zones with clefts of dissolved urate crystals are surrounded by mononuclear phagocytes and some multinuclear giant cells. H&E, ×220

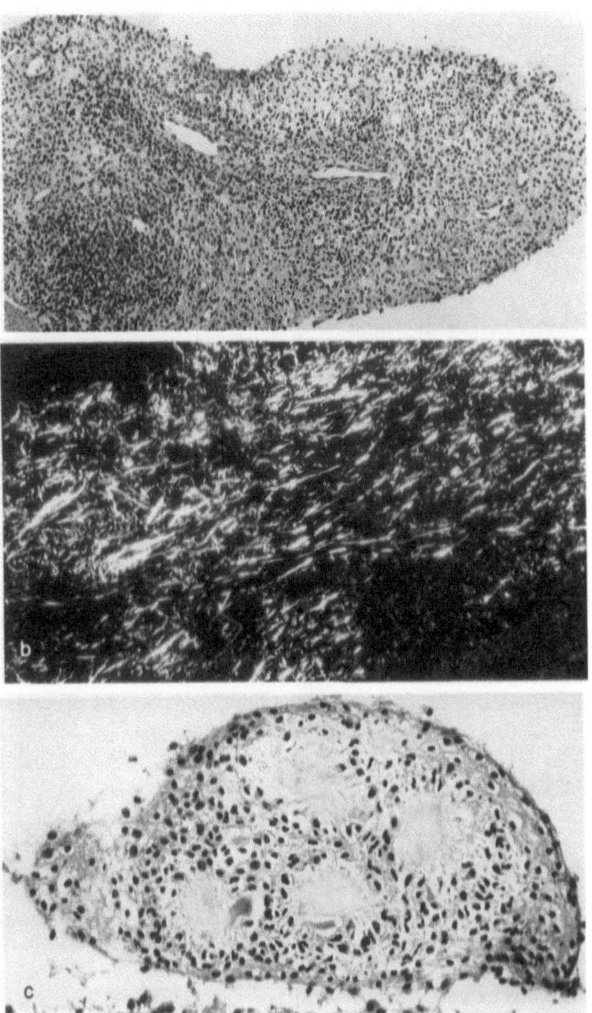

Fig. 19 a–c. Gout or not? (alcohol-dehydrated tissue). **a** Appearance of a synovial villus in the conventional H&E-stained section: lympho-plasmocytic infiltration of the synovial membrane. ×85. **b** Unstained section of alcohol-dehydrated tissue with demonstration of urate crystals under polarized light. ×220. **c** In a deeper section the occurrence of a synovial villus with small urate granulomata. H&E, ×220

destroy cortical bone and invade the subchondral bone under the preserved cartilage (Fig. 17).

As is the case with the synovial tissue, *tendons* may also become involved either by the interstitial or the synovial fluid. According to Hankin et al. (1985), traumatisation of the tendons influences the location of the urate deposits. Morphologically, nodules of urate can be observed inside the tendons (Uehlinger 1976; Mahoney et al. 1981).

Bursae are often involved (Zöllner 1990) – from an investigation on chronic bursitis, Canoso and Yood (1979) concluded that about 20% of cases of this disease are due to gout. The olecranon and prepatellar bursae are most usually affected. Pathologists regulary observe operation specimens of bursae with urate granulomata (Fig. 18a, b), indicating clinically "undiagnosed" gout. In advanced cases, the bursa is transformed into a huge nodule of "chalky" urate deposits surrounded by fibrous strands (Fig. 18c). Histologically, the characteristic granulomata are present (Fig. 18d).

Non-articular tophi may occur in different areas of the human body (Table 1). However, only rarely have histological investigations been done on them – this is especially true for those of the ear. Whether the initial urate deposits occur in the elastic cartilage or in the subcutaneous tissue has not been investigated.

If gout is regarded under the aspect of a pathological-morphological diagnosis, it can be stated that in most instances it is easy to diagnose the disease, especially if the tissue is dehydrated in alcohol and not fixed in formalin. Sometimes, diagnostic problems may arise when histological sections, even from alcohol-dehydrated tissues, are stained by the conventional H&E method. This situation may be shown by the following brief case report. A synovial biopsy from a 48-year-old patient, dehydrated in alcohol, was investigated for sodium urate or calcium dihydrate pyrophosphate deposits. From the conventionally stained histological slide, the diagnosis "chronic arthritis suspectable of a rheumatoid disease" was stated (Fig. 19a). One histological slide, unstained and mounted in Eukitt, that was not available for the pathologist at work, exhibited a fibrinous exudate with urate crystals under polarized light (Fig. 19b). Furthermore, the deeper sections contained synovial villi with characteristic granulomata (Fig. 19c). From this observation, it may be deduced that unstained sections of alcohol-dehydrated, paraffin-embedded tissue with preservation of the crystals should also be used for diagnostic purposes.

References

Agudelo CA, Schumacher HR (1973) The synovitis of acute gouty arthritis. Hum Pathol 4: 265–279

Brogsitter AM (1926) Histopathologie der Gelenkgicht. Dtsch Arch Klin Med 153: 257–326

Bunim JJ, McEwen C (1940) Tophus of the mitral valve in gout. Arch Pathol 29: 700–704

Canoso JJ, Yood RA (1979) Reaction of superficial bursae in response to specific disease stimuli. Arthritis Rheum 22: 1361–1364

Das De S (1988) Intervertebral disc involvement in gout: brief report. J Bone Joint Surg [Br] 70: 671

Farebrother DA, Hatfield P, Simmonds HA, Cameron JS, Jones AS, Cadenhead A (1975) Experimental crystal nephropathy (one year study in the pig). Clin Nephrol 4: 243–250

Garrod AB (1859) The nature and treatment of gout and rheumatic gout. Walton and Maberly, London

Gieseking R (1972) Elektronenoptische Befunde am Gichttophus. Therapiewoche 22: 108–113

Hankin FM, Mayhew DE, Coapman RA, Snedden M, Schneider LH (1985) Gouty infiltration of a flexor tendon simulating rupture. Clin Orthop 194: 172–175

Hirohata K, Morimoto K, Kimura H (1981) Ultrastructure of bone and joint disease. Igaku-Shoin, Tokyo New York

Kersley GD, Mandel L, Jeffrey MR (1950) Gout – An unusual case with softening and subluxation of the first cervical vertebra and splenomegaly. Ann Rheum Dis 9: 282–304

Kirkpatrick CJ, Mohr W, Haferkamp O (1981) The effect of soluble sodium urate on the proliferation and proteoglycan synthesis of lapine articular chondrocytes in monolayer culture. Rheumatol Int 1: 131–133

Linnane JW, Burry AF, Emmerson BT (1981) Urate deposits in the renal medulla. Prevalence and associations. Nephron 29: 216–222

Mahoney PG, James PD, Howell CJ, Swannell AJ (1981) Spontaneous rupture of the achilles tendon in a patient with gout. Ann Rheum Dis 40: 416–418

Martinez-Cordero E, Barreira-Mercado E, Katona G (1986) Eye tophi deposition in gout. J Rheumatol 13: 471–472

Mohr W (1984) Arthropathien. In: Doerr W, Seifert G, Uehlinger E (eds) Pathologie der Gelenke und Weichteiltumoren I. Spezielle pathologische Anatomie Band 18/I. Springer, Berlin Heidelberg New York Tokyo (pp 373–547)

Niemi K-M (1977) Panniculitis of the leg with urate crystal deposition. Arch Dermatol 113: 655–656

Palacios-Boix A, Kraus A, Alarcón-Segovia D (1984) Location of tophi at Cushing's striae. J Rheumatol 11: 720–721

Palmer DG, Hogg N, Denholm I, Allen CA, Highton J, Hessian PA (1987) Comparison of phenotype expression by mononuclear phagocytes within subcutaneous gouty tophi and rheumatoid nodules. Rheumatol Int 7: 187–193

Palmer DG, Highton J, Hessian PA (1989) Development of the gout tophus. An hypothesis. Am J Clin Pathol 91: 190–195

Pritzker KPH, Zahn CE, Nyburg SC, Luk SC, Houpt JB (1978) The ultrastructure of urate crystals in gout. J Rheumatol 5: 7–18

Sokoloff L (1957) The pathology of gout. Metabolism 6: 230–243

Traut EF, Knight AA, Szanto PB, Passerelli EW (1954) Specific vascular changes in gout. JAMA 156: 591–593

Uehlinger E (1976) Pathologische Anatomie der Gicht. Verh Dtsch Ges Rheumatol 4: 95–101

Virchow R (1868) Seltene Gichtablagerungen. Virchows Arch 44: 137–138

Zetkin M, Kühtz E-H, Fichtel K (1964) Wörterbuch der Medizin. VEB Verlag Volk
    und Gesundheit, Berlin
Zoller WG, Füeßl HS, Löffler W, Keller C (1985) Gichttophus mit seltener Lokalisa-
    tion. Münch Med Wochenschr 127: 200–201
Zöllner N (1990) Die chronische Gicht: In: Zöllner N (ed) Hyperurikämie; Gicht und
    andere Störungen des Purinhaushaltes. Springer, Berlin Heidelberg New York
    London Paris Tokyo Hongkong Barcelona (pp 158–168)

Questions and Comments Raised for Discussion

J. T. SCOTT

The slides which were presented are beautiful. I suppose that your illustra-
tions of urate crystals in articular cartilage are consistent with two processes
going on – first, urate damaging cartilage with secondary osteoarthritis and,
secondly, urate becoming deposited in cartilage which is already damaged.

You described a tophus as an inflammatory-induced nodule. While from
the pathological point of view this must be correct, with the presence of
surrounding inflammatory cells, from the clinical point of view a tophus is
usually an indolent structure, producing little in the way of acute inflammation.

R. W. E. WATTS

It seems to me that a particularly fruitful line of research would be to examine
the subclasses of lymphocytes and possibly of other mononuclear cells which
are recruited during the evolution of the inflammatory response to monosodium urate crystals and in tophus formation. Morphology and cell counting
techniques may not be sufficiently sharp tools with which to explain the
differences in the tissue responses to types of crystals which are as diverse in
crystallographic structure as monosodium urate, hydroxy apatite or, indeed,
calcium oxalate dihydrate ("oxalate gout" was not mentioned in the discussion). Perhaps the crystal habit is an important factor as well as their chemical
composition.

K. L. SCHMIDT

What is the histological picture of the enlargement of tophi? Do they grow
due to an increase of the crystallisation foci, by of necrosis or of cellular
proliferation?

4

Questions and Comments Raised for Discussion

M. GONELLA and G. CALABRESE

Chronic gouty nephropathy has been considered so far as a form of chronic tubulointerstitial nephritis, due to long-standing hyperuricemia, often leading to renal failure.

The pathological picture is characterized by sodium urate deposits in the renal interstitium at times presenting as tophi.

Clinically, the condition is as any chronic tubulointerstitial disease with mild urinary abnormalities and impaired tubular functions.

The development and the progression of renal failure, due to chronic gouty nephropathy, have been questioned by recent studies, which pointed out that in most gouty patients the decline of renal function could be attributed to other associated diseases such as arteriosclerosis, hypertension, chronic lead intoxication and preexisting nephropathies.

However, in cases of inherited enzymatic defects (total or partial HGPRT deficiency) or familial juvenile gout, hyperuricemia might be the main cause of progressive renal failure.

In conclusion, whenever hyperuricemia or gout precede or are associated with renal impairment, all the above clinical entities should be considered in the differential diagnosis.

Renal Consequences of Hyperuricemia

M. Gonella and G. Calabrese

The renal consequences of hyperuricemia include:
- Acute uric acid nephropathy, due to the precipitation of uric acid crystals within the tubule lumina, which usually occurs because of acute overproduction of uric acid in patients on cytotoxic therapy for lympho- and myeloproliferative disorders.
- Uric acid nephrolithiasis, which implies the formation of uric acid stones in the urinary tract due to hyperuricosuria and/or acid urine, with or without hyperuricemia.
- Chronic gouty nephropathy, to which the present chapter is devoted with particular attention to the differential diagnosis.

Chronic gouty nephropathy has been defined so far as a form of chronic tubulointerstitial nephritis because of deposits of sodium urate crystals within the renal interstitium resulting from long-standing hyperuricemia [1–5].

Pathology

The pathological picture found in patients with Lesch–Nyhan syndrome and in those with partial deficiency of hypoxanthine-guanine-phosphoribosyl transferase (HGPRT) can be taken as a model of chronic gouty nephropathy, since in these disorders there are no factors apart from hyperuricemia and hyperuricosuria that may affect the kidney [1].

The sodium urate deposits in the renal interstitium may present as tophi, which usually appear in the medulla as crystal-shaped lacunae (as sodium urate washes out with aqueous fixatives and is preserved with alchol fixatives), surrounded by foreign body giant cells which in turn are surrounded by histiocytes [6]. However, the interstitial tophi are not always found in gout [6], and they were also described at autopsy in gout-free patients [4, 7]. The existence of glomerular lesions (fibrillar thickening of the capillary basement membrane and increased nuclei in capillary loops) described in gouty nephropathy [8] is attributed by most authors to concomitant factors such as ischemia, chronic infection, and obstruction [3, 9, 10].

Although questioned as a specific entity, chronic gouty nephropathy has been classified as a chronic tubulointerstitial disease, without any specific clinical hallmark. As such, asymptomatic urinary abnormalities (mild proteinuria lower than 1 g/day, microscopic hematuria, and/or leucocyturia) and impaired concentrating ability can occur.

Nowdays, the progression of isolated gouty nephropathy toward renal failure is strongly debated and attributed to other factors, as will be discussed in the following sections.

Pathogenesis

The pathogenesis and even the very existence of chronic gouty nephropathy have been questioned in the past decade because of the results of more recent studies and critical evaluation of previous observations. In 1952, Modern and Meister reported on three patients with gout and renal insufficiency, and they defined this entity as "the kidney of gout" because it was characterized clinically by renal failure, fixed specific gravity, increased azotemia, and, in the single autopsy performed, renal tophi, tubular atrophy, and interstitial fibrosis; however, two of the patients had suffered from severe vascular disease [11]. In a pathological and retrospective autopsy study of 279 patients, Talbott and Terplan tried to define better the correlation between renal lesions and the development of clinical features. They found mainly pyelonephritis scars, intrarenal tophi often surrounded or obscured by stellate scars, arterial sclerosis, and interstitial fibrosis. Furthermore, a correlation was found between the clinical severity of gout and the severity of renal pathology, but with relevant exceptions; moreover, 50% of the patients with severe gout had died from uremia. As pointed out by Beck [12], most of these patients also suffered from coronary artery disease, heart failure, or hypertension other than from severe gout; in addition, minimal clinical evidence of renal impairment was present in a few patients with severe tophaceous gout [2]. Later, Barlow and Beilin performed biopsies in 25 patients with primary gout; they concluded that needlelike urate crystals in the medullary interstitial tissue surrounded by inflammatory cells are the most specific findings in gout nephropathy. However, they noted the presence of nephrosclerosis in almost all the patients studied, whereas this finding was present in only 46% of age-matched controls [3].

New lights on the relationship between hyperuricemia and gouty nephropathy were shed by Yu and Berger [13, 14] and Fessel [15], who carried on between 1973–1982 longitudinal studies on several hundred patients with gout, evaluating the long-term effect on renal function of hyperuricemia, alone or associated with other diseases, and the possible protective action of uric-acid-lowering drugs. They concluded that gout and hyperuricemia alone are not responsible for the decrease of renal function, but rather it is caused by the coexistence of hypertension, vascular disease, or independent nephropathies. These conclusions were confirmed by other authors [16, 17].

Differential Diagnosis

Since the existence of chronic gouty nephropathy and its harmful effect on renal function are questioned, as previously discussed, when hyperuricemia precedes or is associated with renal failure, other diagnoses should be considered (Table 1).

– *Chronic lead intoxication* [17–22], which is known to cause hyperuricemia and progressive renal failure. The diagnosis of lead poisoning can be ascertained by careful history taking, signs and subjective symptoms, and laboratory abnormalities.

– *Hypertension.* Apart from the known epidemiological association between gout and hypertension, hypertensive states can affect renal urate handling [23, 24]. In fact, a common etiological factor could be the high level of angiotensin II and norepinephrine which increase the filtration fraction, thereby enhancing urate reabsorption [23–27]. Therefore, when hypertension and hyperuricemia are associated and precede renal impairment, hypertension must be considered as a possible cause responsible for the progression of renal failure.

– *Nephropathies and hyperuricemia.* In cases of hyperuricemia disproportionate to renal function, the possible existence and the nature of a primary nephropathy must be considered. In fact, although the increase of plasma uric acid concentration is not proportional to the reduction of glomerular filtration because of adaptive tubular mechanisms and of increased intestinal uricolysis [28, 29], a wide range of plasma uric acid levels was noted to be associated with a similar degree of renal function. As a matter of fact, uricemia was found to be disproportionately high when compared with other nephropathies under the following conditions: (a) acute and chronic glomerulonephritis [30, 31], in which an urate overproduction or a specific defect in urate excretion can be postulated ; (b) preeclampsia or eclampsia, in which the degree of hyperuricemia was found to be directly correlated with the severity of glomerular lesions [32]; (c) polycystic and medullary cystic disease of the kidney, which are associated with more severe hyperuricemia and occasionally gout [33–35]; (d) hemolytic uremic syndrome, in which hyperuricemia, attributed to acute cell lysis, was shown to be a constant feature [36] – in addition, it was postulated that the frequent occurrence of oligoanuria in this syndrome may be due to acute urate nephropathy (uric acid precipitation in collecting ducts) superimposed on the acute glomerulopathy [37, 38]; (e) a possible association between hyperuricemia or gout and lupus nephritis has been described in young women [39], in whom otherwise hyperuricemia is rare. Therefore, in patients with renal failure and disproportionate hyperuricemia, the existence of the above primary or secondary nephropathies must be excluded because they per se lead to progressive renal failure.

– *Type I glycogen storage disease*, caused by glucose-6 phosphatase deficiency, determines growth retardation, hepatomegaly, lactic acidemia, hyperuricemia with the possible complication of gouty arthritis [40], and, as re-

Table 1. Diagnostic approaches to concomitant hyperuricemia and/or gout and progressive nephropathy

Underlying disease	Epidemiology	Clinical features	Laboratory findings
Chronic lead intoxication	Professional exposure; occult sources	Peripheral neuropathy, ataxia, anemia, abdominal pain, headache	Blood lead level >25 µg/dl Increased urinary levels after EDTA mobilization test Microcytic hypochromic anemia Prolonged nerve conduction time Renal glycosuria and aminoaciduria
Hypertension	Middle age in essential HP; any age in secondary HP	Signs and symptoms related to HP and/or to the underlying disease in secondary HP	Related to underlying disease in secondary HP Mild urinary abnormalities
Primary or secondary nephropathies	Variable according to specific nephropathy		
Type I glycogen storage disease	Recessive autosomic; early manifestation; gout and renal complication in the long-term	Growth retardation, hepatomegaly, signs of acidosis, eruptive xanthomas	Glucose-6 phosphatase deficiency in hepatic cells Hypoglycemia, hyperlipemia Lactic acidosis Marked proteinuria Microscopic hematuria Focal segmental glomerulosclerosis
HGPRT deficiency	X-linked recessive inheritance; young males	Total deficiency: Lesch–Nyhan syndrome Partial deficiency: gout, renal failure, kidney stones	Total or partial defect of HGPRT in lysed RBCs Increased adenine phosphoribosyltransferase activity in lysed RBCs Increased phosphoribosyl-pyrophosphate levels Microscopic or gross hematuria Urinary urate crystals
Familial juvenile gout	Strong family history; young age; in both sexes	Gouty arthritis, possible associated malformations, possible mild jaundice	Serum Uric Acid disproportion-ately high for sex, age, and GFR Possible severe reduction of urinary concentration capacity Possible signs of hemolytic anemia

HP, hypertension; EDTA, ethylendiamine tetraacetic acid; HGPRT, hypoxanthine-guanine phosphoribosyl transferase; GFR, glomerular filtration rate; RBC, red blood cell

cently pointed out, renal failure with an accompanying histological picture of focal segmental glomerulosclerosis in a few patients [41].

– *Deficiency of HGPRT* (the enzyme that catalyzes the salvage of the purine bases hypoxanthine and guanine to inosine monophosphate and guanine monophosphate) produces a broad spectrum of clinical signs depending on the severity of the enzyme defect: The complete defect causes the Lesch–Nyhan syndrome, whereas a partial defect can lead to, in the absence of neurological involvement, hyperuricemia, gout, renal failure, and kidney stones [42–44]. In these patients, chronic uric acid overproduction leads to hyperuricosuria in addition to marked hyperuricemia. The contemporary presence of intratubular uric acid and interstitial urate deposits observed in these patients has been explained by two hypotheses: According to the first one, crystal deposition in the tubules leads to intratubular obstruction with a resulting decline in renal function, which would cause a further rise in plasma uric acid and deposition of microtophi in the interstitium [45]; the second hypothesis postulates that uric acid crystals may erode from the tubules into the interstitium, subsequently transforming into sodium urate [46]. The diagnosis of partial deficiency is based on the finding of low levels of the enzyme in lysed and intact red cells [44].

– *Familial juvenile gout.* The coexistence of juvenile gout and progressive renal failure has been documented by many authors [5, 47–52]. In the kindred, a strong family history was described with gout affecting one or more members in the first decades of life, irrespective of sex, and a frequently rapid decline of renal function. The relationship between hyperuricemia and/or gout and renal failure is somehow controversial and probably different in the various suffererers. In fact, some reports considered a long-standing hyperuricemia responsible for the decrease of renal function; they supported this hypothesis with pathological findings of focal or diffuse interstitial fibrosis and chronic inflammatory cells and tubular atrophy, even in the absence of urate crystals, except in one case [49–51, 53, 54]. In describing a similarly affected relative, other authors suggested that, at least sometimes, there is an interstitial nephropathy inherited as an autosomal dominant trait and leading to renal failure, and hyperuricemia would be an indicator of primary tubular involvement [5]. Apart from the cause and effect relationship between hyperuricemia and renal failure, the coexistence of these features in subjects within the third decade of age, a strong family history, a similar incidence in both sexes, the finding of a plasma uric acid level disproportionately high for age and sex, and a subnormal uric acid clearance rate relative to the glomerular filtration rate (FEur) may suggest the diagnosis of familial juvenile gout [52].

Conclusion

Although urate crystal deposits can occur in patients with gout or sustained hyperuricemia, the development of renal failure is uncommon, except probably in a few patients with severe hyperuricemia from inherited disorders. The decrease of renal function in patients with gout may usually be attributed to other associated diseases such as vascular disease, hypertension, chronic lead intoxication, or preexisting nephropathy.

References

1. Emmerson BT, Row PG (1975) An evaluation of the pathogenesis of the gouty kidney. Kidney Int 8: 65
2. Talbott JH, Terpaln KL (1960) The kidney in gout. Medicine 39: 405
3. Barlow KA, Beilin LS (1968) Renal disease in primary gout. Q J Med 37: 79
4. Linnane JW, Burry AF, Emmerson BT (1981) Urate deposits in the renal medulla. Nephron 29: 216
5. Leumann EP, Wegman W (1983) Familial nephropathy with hyperuricemia and gout. Nephron 34: 51
6. Zollinger HU, Mihatsch MJ (1978) Enzymopathic and metabolic renal disease. In: Zollinger HU, Mihatsch MJ (eds) Renal pathology in biopsy. Springer, Berlin Heidelberg New York, p 465
7. Verger D, Leroux-Robert C, Ganter P, Richet G (1967) Les tophus goutteux de la medullaire renale des uremiques chroniques. Nephron 4: 356
8. Gonik HC, Rubini ME, Gleason IO, Sommers SC (1965) The renal lesions in gout. Ann Intern Med 62: 667
9. Heptinstall RB (1983) Diabetes mellitus and gout. In: Heptinstall RH (ed) Pathology of the kidney, 3rd ed. Little, Brown and Company, Boston Toronto, p 1438
10. Pardo V, Perez-Stable E, Fisher ER (1968) Ultrastructural studies in hypertension: III Gouty nephropathy. Lab Invest 18: 143
11. Modern FWS, Meister L (1952) The kidney of gout, a clinical entity. Med Clin North Am 36: 941
12. Beck LH (1986) Requiem for gouty nephropathy. Kidney Int 30: 280
13. Yu T, Berger L (1975) Renal disease in primary gout: a study of 253 gout patients with proteinuria. Semin Arthritis Rheum 4: 293
14. Berger L, Yu T (1975) Renal function in gout. An analysis of 524 gouty subjects including long-term follow-up studies. Am J Med 59: 605
15. Fessel WJ (1979) Renal outcomes of gout and hyperuricemia. Am J Med 67: 74
16. Reif MC, Constantiner A, Levitt MF (1981) A vanishing syndrome. N Engl J Med 304: 535
17. Porter G (1983) Gouty nephropathy. Factor finction? Am J Kidney Dis 2: 553
18. Batuman V, Maesaka JK, Haddad B, Wedeen RP (1981) The role of lead in gout nephropathy. N Engl J Med 304: 520
19. Wedeen RP, Batuman V (1983) Tubulointerstitial nephritis induced by heavy metals and metabolic disturbances. In: Contran RS (ed) Tubulointerstitial nephropathies, Churchill Livingstone, New York, p 211 (Contemporary Issue in Nephrology, vol 10)
20. Emmerson BT (1968) Clinical differentation of primary gout from lead gout. Arch Rheum 11: 623
21. Yu TF (1983) Lead nephropathy and gout. Am J Kidney Dis 2: 555

22. Cledes J, Allain P, Guillodo MP, Herve JP (1990) Acute gouty arthritis (AGA) in chronic renal failure (CRF): value for diagnosis of increased lead burden (ILB). Abstract EDTA-ERA 5–8 Sept, Vienna, p 74
23. Cannon PJ, Stason WB, Demartini FE etn PJ, Stason WB, Demartini FE et al. (1966) Hyperuricemia in primary and renal hypertension. N Engl J Med 275: 457
24. Brunner HR, Laragh JH, Baer L et al. (1972) Essential hypertension: Renin and aldosterone, heart attack and stroke. N Engl J Med 286: 441
25. Ferris TF, Gorden P (1968) Effect of angiotensin and norepinephrine upon urate clearance in man. Am J Med 44: 359
26. Simon NM, Smucker JE, O'Conor JVVr, Del Greco F (1969) Differential uric acid excretion in essential and renal hypertension. Circulation 39: 121
27. Berger L, Yu TF, Kupfer AS, Gutman AB (1964) Effects of reducing renal arterial blood pressure by ballon catheter on urate excretion in the dog. Proc Soc Exp Biol Med 115: 58
28. Steele TH, Rieselbach RE (1975) Renal urate excretion in normal man. Nephron 14: 21
29. Rieselbach RE, Steele TH (1975) Intrinsic renal disease leading to abnormal urate excretion. Nephron 14: 81
30. Gonella M, Mariani G (1984) Behaviour of serum urate in renal disease of varying etiology. In: Be Bruyn CHMM, Simmonds HA, Muller MM (eds) Purien metabolism in man. Plenum Press, New York, p 205 (Advances in experimental medicine and biology, vol 165 A)
31. Mukhin NA, Serov UV, Maksimov NA et al. (1985) Hyperuricemic variant of latent glomerulonephritis. Abstract ter Arkh 57 (6): 43
32. Emmerson BT, Ravenscroft PJ (1975) Abnormal renal urate homeostasis in systemic disorders. Nephron 14: 62
33. Rivera JV, Martinez-Maldonado M, Ramirez de Azellano G, Ehrlich L (1965) Association of hyperuricemia and polycystic kidney disease. Bol Assoc Med P R 57: 251
34. Newcombe DS (1973) Gouty arthritis and polycystic kidney disease. Ann Intern Med 79: 605
35. Thompson GR, Weiss JJ, Goldman RT, Rigg GA (1978) Familial occurrence of hyperuricemia, gout, and medullary cystic disease. Arch Intern Med 138: 1614
36. Kaplan RS, Thomson PN (1976) Hyperuricemia in the hemolytic-uremic syndrome. Am J Dis Child 130: 854
37. O'Regan, Rousseau E (1988) Hemolytic uremic syndrome: urate nephropathy superimposed on an acute glomerulopathy? An hypothesis. Clin Nephrol 30: 207
38. Rousseau E, Blasis N, O'Regan S (1990) Decreased necessity for dialysis with loop diuretic therapy in hemolytic uremic syndrome. Clin Nephrol 34: 22
39. Frocht A, Leek JC, Robbins DL (1987) Gout and hyperuricaemia in systemic lupus erythematosus. Br J Rheum 26: 303
40. Kolb FO, De Lalla OF, Gofman JW (1955) The hyperlipemia in disorders of carbohydrate metabolism: serial lipoprotein studies in diabetic acidosis with xanthomatosi and in glycogen storage disease. Metabolism 4: 310
41. Chen YT, Coleman RA, Scheinman JI et al. (1988) Renal disease in Type I glycogen storage disease. N Engl J Med 318: 7
42. Nyhan WL (1982) Inborn errors of purine metabolism. In: Cockburn F, Gitzelmann R (eds) Inborn errors of metabolism in humans. MPT press, Lancaster, p 13
43. Emmerson BT, Thompson L (1973) The spectrum of hypoxanthine-guanine phosphoribosiltransferase deficiency. Q J Med 166: 423

44. Cameron JS, Simmonds HA, Webster DR et al. (1984) Problems of diagnosis and in vitro enzyme instability in an adolescent with hypoxanthine-guanine phosphoribosiltransferase deficiency presenting in acute renal failure. In: De Bruyn DHMM, Simmonds HA, Muller MM (eds) Purine metabolism in man. Plenum Press, New York, p 7 (Advances in experimental medicine and biology, vol 165 A

45. Kelton J, Kellcy WN, Holmes EW (1978) A rapid method for the diagnosis of acute acid nephropathy. Arch Intern Med 138: 612

46. Cameron JS, Simmonds HA (1981) Uric acid and the kidney. J Clin Pathol 34: 1245

47. Duncan H, Dixon A St.J. (1960) Gout, familial hyperuricemia, and renal disease. Q J Med 29: 127

48. Van Goor W, Kooiker CJ, Doorhout Mees EJ (1971) An unusual form of renal disease associated with gout and hypertension. J Clin Pathol 24: 354

49. Simmonds HA, Warren DJ, Cameron JS et al. (1980) Gout and renal failure in young women. Clin Nephrol 14: 176

50. Massari PU, Hsu CH, Barnes RV et al. (1980) Familial hyperuricemia and renal disease. Arch Intern Med 140: 680

51. Richmond JM, Kincaid-Smith P, Whitworth JA, Becker GS (1981) Familial urate nephropathy. Clin Nephrol 16: 163

52. Calabrese G, Simmonds HA, Cameron JS, Davies PM (1990) Precocious familial gout with reduced fractional urate clearance and normal purine enzymes. Q J Med 75: 441

53. Warren DJ, Simmonds HA, Gibson T, Naik RB (1981) Familial gout and renal failure. Arch Dis Childhood 56: 699

54. Westberg NG, Rosen E, Waldenstrom J (1979) Recessive x-linked hyperuricemia with gout and renal damage, normal activity of hypoxanthine phosphoribosiltransferase and resistance to azaguanin. Acta Med Scan 205: 163

Urate and Uric Acid Crystal Reactions Within the Kidney – Clinical and Experimental Studies

B. T. EMMERSON

Introduction

Gout Is Not a Single Disease

It is difficult to define the complications of gout because gout is not a single disease entity, and there will often be multiple factors contributing to the development of complications. Accordingly, it should not be expected that such complications will have a uniform pattern.

The relationship of gout with renal disease is further complicated by the fact that the renal disease can be primary and the gout secondary, whereas some types of gout may lead to secondary renal disease. Other types of gout may have no relationship to renal disease whatsoever.

Complications Are Not Uniform

We would all agree that since the development of allopurinol the frequency of renal disease in patients with gout has declined. That it was not always so is attested to by the publications prior to the development of allopurinol. Even in 1966, crystals for X-ray diffraction studies could be found in the kidneys of 6 of 11 patients with gout who were studied (Seegmiller and Frazier 1966). However, although the frequency of renal disease in these patients has declined, its importance has not diminished. The reasons for this will be considered.

Relationship of Gout and Renal Disease

Uric Acid Nephropathy in Tumour Lysis

Acute uric acid nephropathy is still a common problem in the tumour lysis syndrome. Such patients are seen regularly in our major hospitals, presenting with acute renal failure which can often be prevented by allopurinol administration and an alkaline diuresis. However, even with this prophylaxis, some degree of acute renal failure is not uncommon following chemotherapy of malignancies with its nucleoprotein degradation.

Acute Uric Acid Nephropathy in Primary Over-producers of Urate

Patients with urate over-production due to hypoxanthine phosphoribosyl transferase (HPRT) deficiency may present clinically with acute renal failure which, if it is recognised, is also reversible by an alkaline diuresis (Emmerson et al. 1976). This occurs occasionally in adult life, but it can also arise in infancy as a child several months old may develop acute renal failure (Batch et al. 1984). In some cases, this progresses to chronic renal insufficiency, whereas in others, it appears to be completely reversed. This picture fits with an acute uric acid crystal nephropathy with obstruction of tubules and collecting ducts by the crystals (Emmerson and Thompson 1973), and the potential for this exists whenever conditions within the renal tubule are such as to promote crystal formation.

Clinical Co-existence

Gout and renal disease still co-exist clinically. Patients are seen in whom both entities occur together at an early stage. Some patients have renal insufficiency at the time of their first attack of gout. Thus, in view of the differing management required if the condition is a primary uric acid abnormality rather than a primary renal disease, it is important to be able to differentiate between them.

Critical Factors Determining Crystal Deposition Within the Kidney

It seems particularly important to consider mechanisms whereby uric acid and gout can cause kidney disease, and I shall be provocative and propose several hypotheses in order to stimulate discussion. I would also like to highlight certain features which I feel are basic to our understanding of the role of urate and uric acid crystals in inducing or being associated with kidney disease.

Urate Gradient in the Medulla

In considering crystal deposits within the kidney, it is important to recognise that, just as there is an increase in sodium and urea concentrations in the renal papilla, a similar gradient can exist for uric acid between the renal cortex, the medulla and the papilla (Epstein and Pigeon 1964). This implies that the urate concentration increases in the collecting duct as the urine passes from the distal convoluted tubule to the renal pelvis.

Silent Renal Microtophi in the Medulla

The observations of Verger et al. (1967), Ostberg (1968) and Linnane et al. (1981) have shown that microtophi may often be found at autopsy in the renal medulla. They were present in 25% of kidneys with pre-existing, non-gouty renal disease and also in some patients with a history of gout. In some cases, as in coroner's autopsies of deaths due to acute trauma, there was no association with any other recognisable factor. It would be of great interest to know whether the prevalence of medullary microtophi is greater in more tropical areas and less in colder climes. Perhaps the only clue we have is that they seem to be less common in people with diabetes, suggesting that the associated diuresis might reduce its frequency. More research is needed on this phenomenon.

Differentiation of Gout Secondary to Primary Renal Disease from Renal Disease Secondary to Primary Gout

It is quite clear that gout can be associated with secondary renal disease (although less commonly in the past 20 years), and there is also clear evidence that renal disease can be complicated by gout, although this type of gout is often not severe clinically and is usually most troublesome when the renal disease is mild. In determining the interrelationship of gout and renal disease in a patient, it is vital to recognise these two possibilities. One of the useful parameters in determining the prime abnormality is to evaluate which came first chronologically (Emmerson, et al. 1980).

Differentiation of Urate from Uric Acid Crystals Within the Kidney

X-ray diffraction studies have been undertaken to identify the nature of the crystal deposits in the kidneys of patients with gout and of those with acute leukaemia (Seegmiller and Frazier 1966). They showed that the crystals in the former were of monosodium urate monohydrate and were principally deposited in the renal interstitium. In acute leukaemia, the crystals were of uric acid and were deposited within the lumina of the renal tubules. This has been confirmed subsequently. Nonetheless, the fundamental distinction between these two types is vital. The needle-shaped urate crystals tend to form at a physiological pH, whereas the more amorphous uric acid crystals occur at a lower pH, as found in urine and tubular fluid.

Urate/Uric Acid Crystal Nephropathy Should Be Differentiated from Gouty Renal Disease

The deposition of urate crystals leads to a cellular reaction with the formation of a microtophus, and this can occur in the renal interstitium just as in any other tissue. However, we would do well to ask whether there is any mechanism whereby uric acid can induce renal disease other than by the formation of crystals (the only possibility which has been postulated so far has involved platelet adhesiveness and that has not been well substantiated). If there is no other mechanism operating, these conditions should be named "urate crystal nephropathy" and "uric acid crystal nephropathy". The term hyperuricaemic nephropathy should be abandoned because, if hyperuricaemia does induce renal disease (and the evidence for this is poor), it can do so only through the formation of crystals of urate or uric acid.

It is important also to recognise that the factors causing urate/uric acid crystal formation within the kidney are essentially the same as those in other tissues (namely the concentration of urate, the concentration of sodium, the pH at the site and the presence or absence of inhibitors of crystallisation). In view of the increased medullary concentration of both urate and sodium and the concurrent acidification of the urine, there is a potentially greater risk of urate/uric acid crystal formation within the kidney than in other tissues or organs. Indeed, it is perhaps surprising that there is not greater damage to the renal papilla from urate/uric acid crystal deposition than is seen.

Mechanisms Whereby Urate/Uric Acid Crystals Can Induce Renal Disease

How do these crystals produce damage to the kidney? Dr. Gonella referred to two hypotheses but I could believe that both hypotheses are correct; they are not inconsistent nor alternative. It seems likely that interstitial microtophi should be able to form in the renal interstitium if the urate concentration there is high enough. Likewise, it is known that uric acid crystals form readily within the renal tubules, and that in an acute uric acid nephropathy due to urate over-production, there is an acute reaction within the kidney which can lead to renal damage. Uric acid crystals can pass into the cytoplasm of these renal cells (Kanwar and Manaligod 1975), and they will react with them and form phagolysosomes within the renal tubular lining cells. They can also probably pass through the tight junctions between the tubular cells. This crystal/cell reaction induces the release of vasodilatory prostaglandins and probably chemotactic factors, so that there is good reason to believe that an interstitial inflammatory response can occur to uric acid crystals which originated within the tubular lumen. This is illustrated by some of the reactions between Madin-Darby canine kidney cells in culture and uric acid and urate crystals (Emmerson et al. 1990).

References

Batch JA, Riek RP, Gordon RB, Burke JR, Emmerson BT (1984) Renal failure in infancy due to over-production of urate. Aust NZ J Med 14: 852–854
Emmerson BT (1973) Chronic lead nephropathy. Kidney Int 4: 1–5
Emmerson BT, Row PG (1975) An evaluation of the pathogenesis of the gouty kidney. Kidney Int 8: 65–71
Emmerson BT, Thompson L (1973) The spectrum of hypoxanthine-guanine phosphoribosyltransferase deficiency. Q J Med 42: 423–40
Emmerson BT, Gordon RB, Johnson LA (1976) Urate kinetics in hypoxanthine-guanine phosphoribosyltransferase deficiency: their significance for the understanding of gout. Q J Med 177: 49–61
Emmerson BT, Stride PJ, Williams G (1980) The clinical differentiation of primary gout from primary renal disease in patients with both gout and renal disease. Adv Exp Med Biol 122 A: 9–13
Emmerson BT, Cross M, Osborne JM, Axelsen RA (1990) Reaction of MDCK cells to crystals of monosodium urate monohydrate and uric acid. Kidney Int 37: 36–43
Epstein FH, Pigeon G (1964) Experimental urate nephropathy: studies of the distribution of urate in renal tissue. Nephron 1: 144–157
Kanwar YS, Manaligod JR (1975) Leukemic urate nephropathy. Arch Pathol 99: 467–472
Linnane JW, Burry AF, Emmerson BT (1981) Urate deposits in the renal medulla: prevalence and associations. Nephron 29: 216–222
Ostberg Y (1968) Renal urate deposits in chronic renal insufficiency. Acta Med Scand 183: 197–201
Seegmiller JE, Frazier PD (1966) Biochemical considerations of the renal damage of gout. Ann Rheum Dis 25: 668–672
Verger D, Leroux-Robert C, Ganter P, Richet G (1967) Presence and role of gouty tophi in the renal medulla of patients with chronic uremia. Nephron 4: 356–370

Uric Acid and Calcium Oxalate Urinary Stone Disease

R. W. E. WATTS

The ease with which uric acid and its salts crystallise from urine and the contribution of uric acid and urate stones to the overall problem of urolithiasis are well known, but uric acid also has a role in relation to calcium oxalate stone disease. Freshly voided urine commonly contains uric acid crystals, especially if it is concentrated and acidic. Calcium oxalate monohydrate and dihydrate crystals can grow epitaxially on uric acid and uric acid dihydrate crystals. Epitaxy is the growth of a crystal in one or more particular orientations on another with a near geometric fit between the respective networks that are in contact. It has also been suggested that colloidal uric acid and urates absorb glycosaminoglycans (mucopolysaccharides), which are among the urinary constituents that normally protect against crystallisation and stone formation.

The urinary uric acid excretion is one of the six urinary risk factors for calcium oxalate urolithiasis. Although it is less important than the low urine volume and oxalate content, it is more important than either the urinary calcium excretion or the average urinary pH and about equal in significance to the urinary excretion of glycosaminoglycans. The higher the urinary uric acid excretion, the greater its importance as a risk factor for calcium oxalate stones. Mixed stones with a core of uric acid identifiable either crystallographically or chemically and sometimes associated with frank hyperuricosuria have been recognised for many years, but the pathogenetic significance of small, possibly temporary changes in urinary uric acid concentration has been less emphasised.

Some authorities recommend the administration of allopurinol to patients with recurrent idiopathic calcium oxalate stones when these have not been prevented by hydration and a low oxalate, low calcium, low purine diet. This should not be a routine measure, but it may be justified in a few very severe and intractable cases when other measures have failed.

A. SIMMONDS

Since the time of Hippocrates it has been known that gout is uncommon in women (3%–7% of cases of primary gout), occurring predominantly in postmenopausal subjects. Table 1 gives details of two unusual cases of untreated hyperuricaemia in women who have experienced a single attack of gout in the past decade.

The first is a carrier for a genetic defect leading to uric acid overproduction: PP-ribose-P synthetase superactivity (PRPS). The second was previously considered to have a "familial renal disease" until gout in 1987 drew

Table 1. Uric acid and creatinine concentrations in 1981 (a) compared with 1989/90 (b)

| Defect | PUA | PCr | UUA | CrCL | UUA/Cr | FE_{ur} |
	μmol/l		mmol/24 h	ml/min		%
PRPS a	450	85	6.0	91	0.55	10.2
b	410	81	7.0	100	0.60	12.0
FJGN a	460	145	–	–	–	–
b	450	449	0.5	10	0.08	8.2
Control	<280		<3.5		<0.3	>10.0

attention to the genetic defect: familial juvenile gouty nephropathy (FJGN). Family investigations revealed hyperuricaemia in two siblings and three of four children, associated with extreme renal urate hypoexcretion (mean FE_{ur} 5.9) and mild to severe renal disease in three of them; the normal renal function in the other two suggests renal urate hypoexcretion precedes renal disease [1]. All hyperuricaemic FJGN subjects are currently treated with allopurinol commensurate with their renal function which, as in earlier kindreds, has seemingly ameliorated the evolution of the renal lesion [2]. This contrasts with the progression of the propositus to maintenance dialysis in the past decade and the normal renal function in the PRPS carrier over the same period, both untreated. The latter demonstrates that hyperuricaemia and hyperuricosuria per se are not necessarily deterimental to renal function.

1. Moro F, Ogg C, Cameron JS, Simmonds HA, Duley JA, McBride MB, Davies PM (1991) Familial juvenile gouty nephropathy with renal urate hypoexcretion preceding renal disease. Clin Nephrol (in press)
2. Cameron JS, Ogg CS, Moro F, Chantler C, Simmonds HA (1990) Precocious familial gout (letter). Lancet ii: 745

J. G. PUIG

Everybody agrees nowadays that most primary gout patients are uric acid underexcretors. So, in some way and from an academic point of view I would say that gout could be defined as a nephropathy that causes a purine metabolic disorder and finally a systemic disorder of which articular manifestations are prominent.

A second point is that most of us would agree that gout by itself is not the condition for a poor renal prognosis. In other words the physiological decline of renal function that occurs with age is similar in gout patients and in the general population.

Third, the syndrome that Anne Simmonds has called "familial juvenile gouty nephropathy" I have named "familial juvenile renal insufficiency and gout." The results of our studies in two families suggest that the inital pathogenic disorder in this syndrome is an autosomal dominant nephropathy characterized by a marked uric acid underexcretion, hyperuricemia and eventual gouty arthritis which progresses to reduction in kidney size and renal insufficiency. Allopurinol treatment in the affected member of both families neither prevented nor halted the progression of renal failure.

R. W. E. Watts

Faced with a patient with advanced renal disease how does one decide whether a patient has hyperuricaemia and gout secondary to primary renal disease or primary hyperuricaemic gout causing sodium urate nephropathy? Renal biopsy has serious limitations because the sodium urate crystals are mainly in the renal medulla and according to B. Emmerson these crystals can occur in normal people.

J. T. Scott

What specific types of defined renal disease especially predispose to hyperuricaemia and gout?

Can we for the moment accept two propositions? First, as pointed out by Bryan Emmerson, the kidney is damaged in hyperuricaemic conditions only by the presence of solid urate or uric acid. Second, a contentious issue, allopurinol delays the progression of renal functional impairment in patients with juvenile familial gout. Now if this is so, the implication is that the nephropathy is due to urate, as originally proposed by Duncan and Dixon. But I'm sure you don't believe this. Are we not dealing with a special form (or forms) of renal disease of unknown aetiology in which hyperuricaemia is a particular feature?

I. Löffler

I do not think that absolute height of urate clearance is the main problem, if one tries to distinguish between the usual form of gout with secondary renal insufficiency on the one hand and familial juvenile gout and nephropathy on the other. In the family we are following in Munich, there is a clear history from youth of a common symptom of interstitial nephritis, namely, increased fluid intake in patients compared with other family members. Thus, hyperuricaemia does not appear to be the first sign of familial juvenile gout and nephropathy at this early stage, but rather one of at least two.

5

Urate Deposition and Stone Formation in the Kidney in Renal Hypouricemia

O. SPERLING

Introduction

Renal hypouricemia is associated with various degrees of hyperuricosuria. This abnormality is the cause of two types of pathological manifestation: uric acid urolithiasis and uric acid nephropathy associated with acute renal failure. In the following, I shall elaborate on the various types of renal hypouricemia, on the mechanism of the renal tubular defect, and on the clinical pathological manifestations.

Differential Diagnosis of Renal Hypouricemia

Hereditary Renal Hypouricemia (isolated defect)

Hereditary renal hypouricemia refers to the condition of increased renal urate clearance caused by a specific (isolated) inborn error of membrane transport for urate in the renal proximal tubule [1].

There are several types of hereditary renal hypouricemia, in which the urate transport defect is only one component in a generalized disturbance of membrane transport. The most common of these is the Fanconi's syndrome [2], including Wilson's disease, cystinosis, galactosemia, and hereditary fructose intolerance. In all of them, uric acid reabsorption in the proximal tubule is decreased along with that of other crystalloid solutes. Another condition associated with renal hypouricemia is the Hartnup syndrome [3].

Acquired Renal Hypouricemia

This type may accompany conditions of extracellular fluid volume expansion, such as inappropriate antidiuretic hormone secretion [4], and various malignancies, e.g., multiple myeloma [5], lymphomas [6], and pulmonary neoplasms [7]. In Hodgkin's disease, the degree of renal urate clearance was found to correlate with the activity of the neoplastic process [7]. Renal hypouricemia may also occur in heavy metal intoxication [8] and following use of outdated tetracyclines [9]. It can also arise in liver diseases, like jaundice [10], in which the degree of renal urate clearance was shown to improve (decrease) with recovery, and cirrhosis [11], in which an inverse correlation was found between serum bilirubin and urate levels.

Components of Renal Handling of Urate in Man

The exact nature of the renal handling of urate in man has not been clarified conclusively. This is due in part to the lack of an animal model in which the renal handling of urate is identical to that in man. Experiments in man were limited to the study of the effects of urate loading [12, 13] and of various drugs [14–16] on uric acid excretion. Important information was furnished by the inborn defects in renal urate reabsorption in man.

Glomerular Filtration of Uric Acid

Urate is probably bound to plasma proteins, the amount of binding being approximately 5%–10% [17, 18]. Urate is freely filtered at the glomerulus [19].

Reabsorption of Uric Acid

In man, the fractional clearance of urate compared with that of inulin or creatinine is about 7%–10%, indicating very efficient reabsorption. In all animals in which urate reabsorption has been localized, including the cebus monkey [20], it was found to occur largely in the proximal tubules. Urate reabsorption is an active transport process. This is evident from the finding in free-flow, micropuncture studies that the ratio between urate concentration in the proximal tubule fluid to that in plasma is less than 1 [21]. There is additional experimental evidence for this [22]. Studies in the rat in vivo and in vesicles in vitro demonstrated that urate reabsorption is inhibited by a number of substances, e. g., probenecid and furosemide, indicating that urate reabsorption is mediated by an anion exchange mechanism.

Secretion of Uric Acid

The original evidence for tubular urate secretion in man was found in 1950 [23] in the first subject with renal hypouricemia, in whom the fractional urate clearance (FC_{ur}) was 1.46. This early demonstration of the bidirectional tubular transport of urate was subsequently augmented by studies in man, in whom the FC_{ur} was increased artificially, by use of urate loading, mannitol

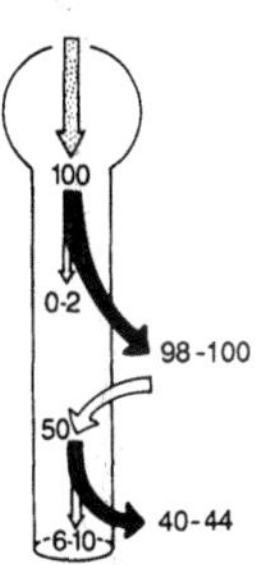

Fig. 1. Model for the renal handling of urate in man. *Stippled arrow* represents filtered urate, *solid arrow* urate reabsorption, and *open arrow* urate secretion or urate remaining in tubular fluid after reabsorption. *Numerical values* indicate hypothetical orders of magnitude of the transport processes. (From Rieselbach and Steele [31]) *American Journal of Medicine*

diuresis, and probenecid, to as great as 1.23 [13]. In man, the exact localization of urate secretion has not been conclusively established. In one study [24], the proximal nephron was found to transport urate to the tubular fluid, whereas the distal nephron was unable to do so. In vivo microperfusion and microinjection studies indicated that similar to the reabsorption of urate, the secretory process is a result of an anion exchange mechanism [25]. An interesting finding in the rabbit is that urate secretion is modulated by a serum protein which affects the basolateral transporter by allosteric modification [26]. This may be taken to suggest that abnormalities in renal urate handling may also reflect primary defects in such modulators of secretion or reabsorption (see below).

Models for Renal Urate Handling in Man

Studies on renal handling of urate in man generated models of a two-, a three-, and finally of a four-component system. The first included glomerular filtration followed by tubular reabsorption [12]. The second one involved in addition the component of secretion [27]. More recently, a fourth component, that of postsecretory reabsorption, was added [28–31] in order to explain the effects of pyrazinamide in some patients or conditions [6, 27], which otherwise, according to the three-component model, could only be interpreted as enhanced tubular secretion of urate. The four-component model (Fig. 1) is comprised of glomerular filtration, early proximal reabsorption, later proximal secretion, and extensive postsecretory reabsorption, which could occur at the same location as the secretion, or separate and distal to it, or both. Recently, a similar model was proposed with the same four components but according to which reabsorption and secretion of urate occur simultaneously along the entire proximal tubule, each at different intensities at the various segments of the tubule [32].

Factors That Affect Renal Handling of Urate in Man

Urate excretion becomes less efficient with age [33, 34], and the mean clearance of urate is 1.2–2.3 ml/min higher in women than men [35].

The extracellular fluid volume (or more precisely, the volume of the effective arterial circulation) is the most dominant factor in renal urate handling. Volume expansion increases urate clearance, whereas contraction decreases it. Presumably, these effects are mediated through alterations in urate reabsorption in the proximal tubule [36, 37].

Many drugs affect renal urate excretion [32, 38]. A biphasic effect was documented for some and suggested for all others [38]. Pyrazinamide, probenecid, phenylbutazone, and salicylate inhibit urate secretion at low doses and urate reabsorption at high doses [27, 39]. Diuretic drugs are initially uricosuric by direct inhibition of urate reabsorption, but their chronic administration is associated with contraction of the extracellular fluid volume, resulting in antiuricosuria [27]. An additional property of some diuretic drugs is their tendency to compete with tubular urate secretion, decreasing further urate excretion [40].

Nature of the Renal Tubular Defect

Increased renal urate clearance could be caused by defective reabsorption or increased secretion. Based on the models of the renal handling of urate in man [28–31], as presented above, five main possibilities of specific abnormalities in active urate transport processes were considered by Sperling [1] as causing renal hypouricemia (Fig. 2).

    A. Total transport defect (no reabsorption and no secretion)
    B. Total reabsorption defect
    C. Presecretory reabsorption defect
    D. Postsecretory reabsorption defect
    E. Increased secretion

According to the three-component model of the renal handling of urate in man ([28–31]; Fig. 1), one may distinguish between the above types of transport defects by use of drugs inhibiting specifically urate reabsorption or secretion. Two drugs, probenecid and pyrazinamide, are employed for the localization of the tubular defect in renal hypouricemia. Probenecid is an inhibitor of the postsecretory reabsorption, and pyrazinamide is an inhibitor of uric acid secretion. For detailed description of the effect of these drugs on uric acid transport in the renal tubule, the reader is referred to a previously published review [1].

The five types would be expected to conform to the following responses of the drugs (Fig. 2). In a total transport defect (type A), FC_{ur} should be about 1, and this value should not be altered by the administration of pyrazinamide or

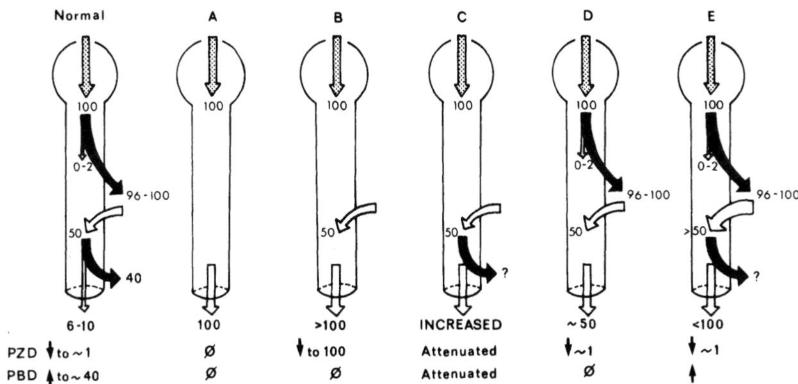

Fig. 2. Five possible defects *(A – E)* that may cause renal hypouricemia and the effects of pyrazinamide *(PZD)* and probenecid *(PBD)* on the fractional clearance of urate. ↑ increase, ↓ decrease (see text for detailed explanation)

probenecid. In a total reabsorption defect but with normal secretion (type B), FC_{ur} should be greater than 1. In such a defect, blocking secretion by pyrazinamide will result in an attenuated decrease in FC_{ur}, which should approach the value of 1. Administration of probenecid will not alter FC_{ur}. In a presecretory reabsorption defect (type C), administration of pyrazinamide will decrease FC_{ur} (which is probably greater than 1), and administration of probenecid will increase this parameter, but both effects will be attenuated. In defective reabsorption at the postsecretory site (type D), FC_{ur} will be smaller than 1 if the amount secreted is less than that filtered. With such a defect, administration of pyrazinamide will decrease FC_{ur} to a normal level, but administration of probenecid will have no effect. In case of a defect manifested in increased secretion (type E), FC_{ur} will probably be smaller than 1 (unless the secretion is increased to such a level that the fraction escaping reabsorption exceeds the amount of filtered urate). In such a defect, the administration of pyrazinamide and of probenecid will result in a normal response.

Type of Defect in Hereditary Renal Hypouricemia (Isolated Defect)

Of the 19 propositi studied for the effects of these drugs [1], 12 could definitely be classified with type C (presecretory reabsorption defect), six with type C or A (total transport defect), and one with type B (total reabsorption defect). None had type D (postsecretory reabsorption defect) or E (increased secretion).

Type of Defect in Other Conditions of Renal Hypouricemia

The pyrazinamide and probenecid tests were done in patients with Fanconi's syndrome [41], Wilson's disease [42], Hodgkin's disease [6], and hyperparathyroidism [43]. Most, if not all, of these subjects could be classified as type D (postsecretory reabsorption defect), which was not found in probands with hereditary isolated renal hypouricemia [1].

The above data may be taken to suggest that type C is the most common (if not the only type) among the subjects with hereditary (isolated) renal hypouricemia, whereas type D (postsecretory reabsorption defect) is most frequent in patients with acquired or hereditary renal hypouricemia associated with a generalized renal tubular reabsorption defect.

Presence of Endogenous Uricosuric Agent as the Primary Defect

In all the above considerations, the existence of an inborn primary renal tubular urate transport defect was presumed. However, caution should be exercised in view of the possibility that the renal tubular abnormalities may be secondary to an irregular metabolite produced elsewhere in the body or to qualitative or quantitative alterations in modulators affecting the urate transport processes. The presence of a humoral uricosuric factor may be possible in some conditions with acquired renal hypouricemia, in which the transitory nature of the defect was demonstrated [6, 44]. Nevertheless, until today, no experimental evidence could be obtained for the presence of a uricosuric agent in the plasma of patients with acquired or hereditary renal hypouricemia [45].

Urate Transport in Nonrenal Tissue of Subjects with Hereditary Renal Hypouricemia

Uric acid transport into erythrocytes was studied in five hypouricemic subjects [46, 47]. In all, urate uptake by the erythrocytes, both total uptake as well as that inhibited by hypoxanthine, was normal. The intestinal absorption of uric acid was gauged in one hypouricemic subject and found similar to that obtained in two control subjects.

Hyperuricosuria

Hyperuricosuria appears to be a constant feature of isolated renal hypouricemia, reflecting diversion of intestinal urate elimination to urinary urate excretion, consequent to the hypouricemia. Uricolysis by intestinal bacteria is responsible for elimination of about 25% of blood uric acid. Blood

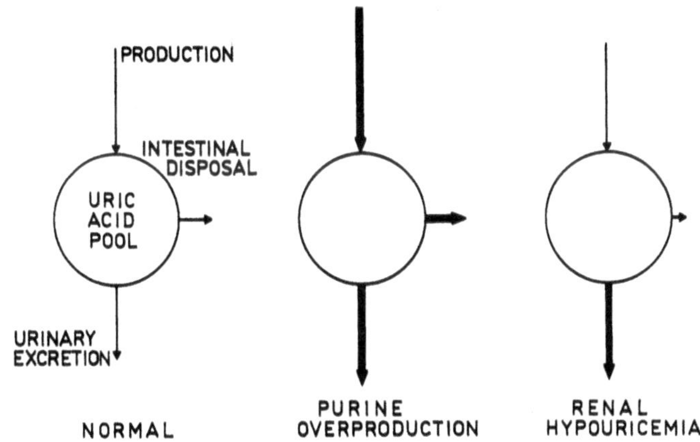

Fig. 3. Effect of hypouricemia on intestinal elimination of uric acid and on urinary uric acid excretion (see text for explanation)

urate level influences the amount of uric acid secreted into the gut. Therefore, in hyperuricemia the fraction of uric acid produced, which is eliminated in the gut, is greater than in normal subjects, whereas in hypouricemia this fraction is markedly smaller. Accordingly, a greater proportion of the uric acid produced leaves the body intact via the kidneys, manifested in hyperuricosuria (Fig. 3). There is no evidence in hypouricemic hyperuricosuric subjects of purine overproduction [48, 49].

Clinical Consequences

Urolithiasis

Five of the 21 propositi studied, with inborn isolated renal hypouricemia [1] had urinary calculi, three uric acid stones, one calcium oxalate stone, and one stone of unidentified composition. For 4 other propositi [50] urolithiasis was present in other family members. The high prevalence of urolithiasis among the subjects with hereditary renal hypouricemia may be explained by the high prevalence of hyperuricosuria. Hyperuricosuria is the most common cause for uric acid/urate supersaturation in urine, and thus it is considered as the underlying cause of the urolithiasis in renal hypouricemia.

Solubility of Uric Acid and Urate in Urine. Uric acid is a weak acid. In the acidic range its solubility increases strongly with increasing pH [51, 52]. The effects of pH and temperature on the solubility were analyzed and found to be in accordance with uric acid being in ideal solution, rather than in a colloidal state [52].

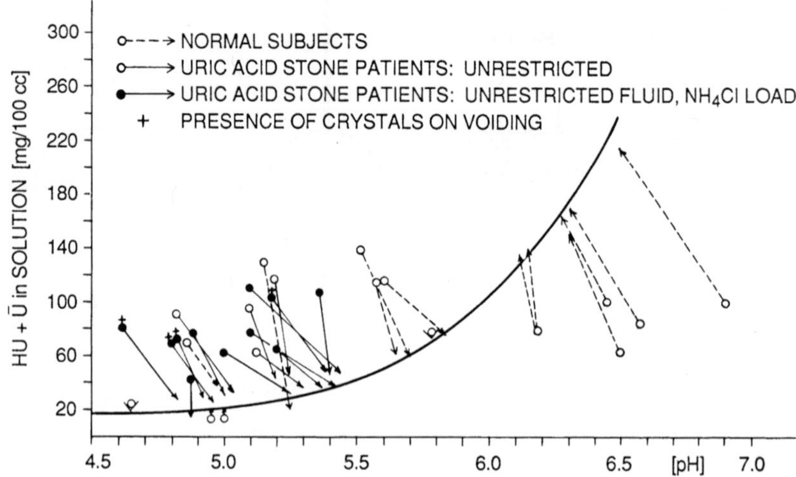

Fig. 4. Uric acid solubility in buffer and urine specimens from normal subjects and patients with idiopathic uric acid lithiasis. *Curve* represents uric acid solubility in buffer solution at equilibrium. Each *arrow* represents one urine equilibration experiment. *Dot at tail of arrow* indicates pH and concentration of uric acid in solution before addition of uric acid crystals. *Head of arrow* represents respective values after equilibration. (From Sperling and De Vries [51])

At a certain solubility product of (U^-) and (Na^+), a new crystalline form, that of the relatively soluble, unstable sodium urate, appears spontaneously, recrystallizing slowly into stable, much less soluble, needle-shaped sodium urate crystals [51]. Since this recrystallization is a slow process, buffer solutions may be supersaturated in regard to these crystals for some time.

The solubility curve for uric acid and sodium urate in urine is identical with that for buffer at physiological salt and urea concentrations ([51]; Fig. 4). Thus, normal urine does not contain any uric-acid-solubilizing substances. Nevertheless, supersaturation frequently occurs in urine, especially at pH below 5.8 [51]. The degree of urine supersaturation in respect to sodium urate is markedly greater than that of uric acid. Indeed, most urines were found to be supersaturated with sodium urate (sodium acid urate; [53]). Fortunately, as discussed above, the spontaneous crystallization of sodium urate is a relatively long process, although high concentrations of sodium and of urate may accelerate it. Studies concerning ammonium acid urate precipitation from urines [54, 55] reveal that in the pH range 6.0–7.5, this crystal could be precipitated only when high concentrations of both urate and ammonium ion were present. Similar to sodium acid urate, the precipitation of ammonium acid urate was also found to be a long process, extending over days.

The state of uric acid supersaturation in normal urine may endure for prolonged periods of time [51]. This is due to the presence in urine of supersaturation-maintaining substances. This property resides in the non-dialyzable urine fraction, specifically in the subfraction constituting only 2%–3% of the total nondialyzable amount and containing a protein with an electrophoretic mobility similar to that of the Tamm–Horsfall mucoprotein ([56]; see [57] for a more complete review on uric acid lithiasis).

Uric Acid Nephropathy

Uric acid nephropathy is distinguished from urate nephropathy in that in the former there is precipitation of uric acid in the collecting tubules, pelvis, or ureter, with subsequent impairment of urine flow, whereas in the latter there is precipitation of monosodium urate in the renal interstitial tissue. Thus, uric acid nephropathy is associated with hyperuricosuria, whereas urate nephro-pathy is associated with hyperuricemia.

Acute uric acid nephropathy is relatively common in the presence of massive uricosuria, such as in the tumor lysis syndrome, but it may also occur in some gouty subjects with excessive purine overproduction, especially in association with inborn errors of metabolism, such as the Lesch–Nyhan syndrome and phosphoribosylpyrophosphate synthetase superactivity.

In view of the prevalence of hyperuricosuria in renal hypouricemia, the possibility of acute uric acid nephropathy in this syndrome should be taken into consideration. Indeed, one such case was reported recently [58]. The patient, a Turkish man residing in Germany, required hemodialysis due to oliguric renal failure. Renal biopsy showed amorphous uric acid crystals in some of the tubular lumina and mild to moderate interstitial inflammation. In this instance the hyperuricosuria was attributed to the increased tubular uric acid secretion.

Very recently, Ishikawa et al. [59] reported mild acute renal failure induced by exercise in three subjects with renal hypouricemia. The clinical manifesta-tions in these patients resembled very much the acute renal failure syndrome described by this group in 1982 [60]. This syndrome, characterized by patchy renal vasoconstriction, is usually mild and nonoliguric, appears in young healthy subjects, and has a good prognosis. There is only a mild to moderate rise in creatine phosphokinase (CPK), suggesting that massive rhabdomyoly-sis does not occur. Ishikawa et al. suggested that in these three patients, the renal failure was caused by the precipitation of uric acid. Nevertheless, this could not be demonstrated.

References

1. Sperling O (1989) Hereditary renal hypouricemia. In: Scriver CR, Beaudet AK, Sly WS and Valle D (eds) The Metabolic Basis of Inherited Disease 6th edition, McGraw-Hill, p 2605
2. Wallis IA, EAGLE RI (1957) The adult Fanconi syndrome. II. Review of eighteen cases. Amer J Med 22: 13–23
3. Baron DN, Dent CE, Harris H, Hard EW, Jebson JB (1956) Hereditary Pellagra-like skin rash with temporary cerebellar ataxia, constant renal aminoaciduria and other bizzare biochemical features. Lancet 271: 421–428
4. Beck IH (1979) Hypouricemia in the syndrom of inappropriate secretion of antidiuretic hormone. New Engl J Med 301: 538–530
5. Smithline N, Kassirer JP, Cohen JJ (1976) Light-chain nephropathy. N Engl J Med 294: 71–74
6. Bennett JS, Bond J, Singer I, Gottlieb AJ (1952) Hypouricemia in Hodgkin's disease. Ann Intern Med 76: 751–756
7. Weinstein B, Irreverre F, Watkin DM (1965) Lung carcinoma, hypouricemia and aminoaciduria. Am J Med 39: 520–526
8. Chisholm JJ Jr, Harrison HAC, Everlein WR, Harrison HE (1955) Amino-aciduria, hypohosphatemia and rickets in lead poisoning. In: Lawson RB, Weech AA, Smyth FS, Kennedy RIJ, Wilson JI, Zuelzer WW (eds) American Journal of Diseases of Children, Chicago American Medical Association, p 159
9. Gross JM (1963) Fanconi syndrome (adult type) developing secondary to the ingestion of outdated tetracycline. Ann Intern Med 48: 523–528
10. Schlosstein L, Kippen I, Bluestone R, Whitehouse MW, Klineberg JR (1974) Association between hypouricemia and jaundice. Ann Rheum Dis 33: 308–312
11. Michelis MF, Warms PC, Fusco RD, Davis BB (1974) Hypouricemia and hyperuricosuria in Laennec cirrhosis. Arch Intern Med 134: 681–683
12. Berliner RW, Hilton JG, Tu TF, Kennedy JR TJ (1950) The renal mechanism for urate excretion in man. J Clin Invest 29: 396–401
13. Gutman AB, Tu TF, Berger L (1959) Tubular secretion of urate in man. J Clin Invest 38: 1778–1781
14. Yu TF, Berger L, Stone DJ, Wolf J, Gutman AB (1957) Effect of pyrazinamide and pyrazinoic acid on urate clearance and other discrete renal functions. Proc Soc Exp Biol (N. Y.) 96: 264–267
15. Yu TF, Berger L, Gutman AB (1961) Suppression of tubular secretion of urate by pyrazinamide in the dog. Proc Soc Exp Biol (N. Y.) 107: 905–908
16. Steele TH, Rieselbach RE (1967) The renal mechanism for urate homeostasis in normal man. Amer J Med 43: 868–875
17. Abramson RG, Levitt MF (1975) Micropuncture study of uric acid in rat kidney. Am J Physiol 228: 1597–1605
18. Wyngaarden JB, Kelley WN (1983) Gout. In: Stanbury JB, Wyngaarden JB, Fredrickson DS, Goldstein JL, Brown MS (eds) The Metabolic Basis of Inherited Disease. McGraw-Hill Book Company, New York, 1983, p 1043
19. Kahn AM, Weinman EJ (1985) Urate transport in the proximal tubule: in-vivo and vesicle studies. Am J Physiol 249: F789–798
20. Roch-Ramel F, Weiner IM (1973) Excretion of urate by the kidney of Cebus monkeys: A micropuncture study. Am J Physiol 224: 1369–1374

21. de Rougemont D, Henchoz M, Roch-Ramel F (1976) Renal urate excretion at various plasma concentrations in the rat: a free-flow micropuncture study. Am J Physiol 231: 387–392
22. Weiner IM, Fanelli GM JR (1975) Renal urate excretion in animal models. Nephron 14: 33–47
23. Praetorius E, Kirk JE (1950) Hypouricemia with evidence for tubular elimination of uric acid. J Lab Clin Med 35: 865–868
24. Podevin R, Ardaillou R, Paillard F, Fontannele J, Richet G (1968) Etude chez l'homme de la cinetique d'apparition dans purine de l'acide urique 2 ^{14}C. Nephron 5: 134–140
25. Weinman EJ, Sansom SC, Steplock DA, Sheth AU, Knight TF, Senekjian HO (1980) Secretion of urate in the proximal convoluted tubule of the rat. Am J Physiol 239: F393–F387
26. Shimomura A, Chonko A, Tanner RM, Edwards R, Grantham JJ (1981) Nature of urate transport in isolated rabbit proximal tubules. Am J Physiol 241: F565–F578
27. Gutman AB, Yu TF (1961) A three-component system for regulation of renal excretion of uric acid in man. Trans Assoc Am Physicians 74: 353–364
28. Steele TH, Boner G (1973) Origins of the uricosuric response. J Clin Invest 52: 1368–1375
29. Steele TH (1973) Urate secretion in man: The pyrazinamide suppression test. Ann Intern Med 79: 734–737
30. Diamond HS, Paolini JS (1973) Evidence for a post-secretory reabsorptive site for uric acid in man. J Clin Invest 52: 1491–1499
31. Rieselbach RE, Steele TH (1974) Influence of the kidney upon urate homeostasis in health and disease. Am J Med 56: 665–675
32. Grantham JJ, Chonko AM (1986) Renal handling of organic anions and cations; metabolism and excretion of uric acid. In: Brenner BM (ed) The Kidney (3rd ed.) Saunders Company, Philadelphia, p 663–700
33. Harkness RA, Nicol AD (1969) Plasma uric acid levels in children. Arch Dis Child 44: 773–778
34. Stapelton FB (1983) Renal uric acid clearance in human neonates. J Pediatr 103: 290–294
35. Wolfson WO, Hunt HJ, Levine E, Gutterman HS, Cohn C, Rosenberg EF, Huddlestun B, Kadota IC (1949) The transport and excretion of uric acid in man V. A sex differential in urate metabolism with a note on clinical and laboratory findings in gouty women. J Clin Endocrinol 9: 749–767
36. Steele TH, Oppenheimer S (1969) Factors affecting urate excretion following diuretic administration in man. Am J Med 47: 563–573
37. Steele TH, Manuel MA, Boner G (1975) Diuretics, urate excretion and sodium reabsorption: A test of acetazolamide and urinary alkalinization. Nephron 14: 48–61
38. Emmerson BT (1978) Abnormal urate excretion associated with renal and systemic disorders, drugs and toxins. In: Kelley WN, Weiner IM (eds) Handbook of Experimental Pharmacology, Uric Acid. Springer-Verlag, Berlin, Vol 51, p 287
39. Yu TF, Gutman AB (1959) Study of the paradoxical effects of salicylate in low, intermediate and high dosage on the renal mechanisms for excretion of urate in man. J Clin Invest 38: 1298–1315
40. Stewart RJ, Chonko AM (1981) Pharmacologic inhibition of urate transport across perfused and non-perfused rabbit proximal straight tubules. Kidney Int 19: 258

41. Meisel AD, Diamond HS (1977) Hyperuricosuria in the Fanconi syndrome. Am J Med Sci 273: 109–115
42. Wilson DB, Goldstein NP (1973) Renal urate excretion in patients with Wilson's disease. Kidney Int 4: 331–336
43. Gibson T, Sims HP, Jimenez SA (1976) Hypouricemia and increased renal urate clearance associated with hyperparathyroidism. Ann Rheum Dis 35: 372–376
44. Weinberger A, Weinberger A, Sperling O, Ben-Bassat M, Kaplan I, Pinkhas J (1977) Increased uric acid clearance in patients with burns. Biomedicine Express 27: 277–278
45. Kay NE, Gotleib AJ (1973) Hypouricemia in Hodgkin's disease: Report of an additional case. Cancer 32: 1508–1511
46. Sperling O, Boer P, Weinberger A, de Vries A (1975) Transport into erythrocytes and intestinal absorption of uric acid in hereditary renal hypouricemia. Biomedicine 23: 157–159
47. Vinay P, Gatterean A, Moulin B, Gougoux A, Lemieux G (1983) Normal urate transport into erythrocytes in familial renal hypouricemia and in Dalmatian dog. Can Med Assoc J 128: 545–549
48. Akaoka I, Nishizawa T, Yano E, Kamatani N, Nishida T, Sasaki S (1977) Renal urate excretion in five cases of hypouricemia with an isolated renal defect of urate transport. J Rheumat 4: 86–94
49. Kawabe K, Muryama T, Akaoka I (1976) A case of uric acid renal stone with hypouricemia caused by tubular reabsorption defect of uric acid. J Urol 116: 690–692
50. Takeda E, Kuroda T, Ito M, Toshima K, Watanabe T, Ito M, Naiko E, Yokota I, Huwang TJ, Miyao M (1985) Hereditary renal hypouricemia in children. J Pediat 107: 71–74
51. Sperling O, de Vries A (1964) Studies on the etiology of uric acid lithiasis. Part II: Solubility of uric acid in urine specimens from normal subjects and patients with idiopathic uric lithiasis. J Urol 92: 331–334
52. Sperling O, Kedem O, de Vries A (1966) Etiologie de la lithiase urique. I. Solubilite de l'acid urique et de l'urate de sodium en solution tampon. Rev Franc d'Etudes Clin et Biol 11: 40–48
53. Coe FL, Strauss AL, Tembe V, Le Dun S (1980) Uric acid saturation in calcium nephrolithiasis. Kidney Int 17: 662–668
54. Teotia M, Sutor J (1971) Crystallization of ammonium acid urate and other uric acid derivatives from urine. Brit J Urol 43: 381–386
55. Teotia M, Teotia SPS (1977) Kidney and bladder stones in India. Postgrad Med J 53: (supp 2) 41–48
56. Sperling O, de Vries A, Kedem O (1965) Studies on the etiology of uric acid lithiasis. IV. Urinary non-dialyzable substances in idiopathic uric acid lithiasis. J Urol 94: 286–292
57. Sperling O (1990) Uric acid nephrolithiasis. In: Wickham JEA and Buck AC (eds) Renal tract stone: Metabolic basis and clinical practice, Churchill Livingstone, London
58. Erley Ch MM, Hirschberg RR, Hoefer W, Schaefer K (1989) Acute renal failure due to uric acid nephropathy in a patient with renal hypouricemia. Klin Wochenschr 67: 308–312
59. Ishikawa I, Sakurai Y, Masuzaki S, Sugishita N, Shinoda A, Shikura N (1990) Exersice-induced acute renal failure in 3 patients with renal hypouricemia. Japanese J Nephrology 32: 923–928

60. Ishikawa I, Onoudi Z, Yuri T et al. (1982) Acute renal failure with severe loin pain and patchy renal vasoconstrictions. In: Eliahou HE (ed) Acute Renal Failure. Libbey, London, p 224

Questions and Comments Raised for Discussion

G. VAN DEN BERGHE

It should be mentioned that there is another condition in which uric acid nephrophathy has been reported, namely respiratory distress syndrome in newborns. In this condition overproduction of uric acid results from anoxia which induces purine catabolism. Although in principle renal clearance of uric acid is high in newborns, the combination of hyperuricosuria and acidosis favours the formation of uric acid crystals, which are very frequently found on autopsy when these babies die.

Acute Renal Insufficiency: Which Mechanisms Are Involved?

R. A. De Abreu

Hyperuricemia has often been noted in the tumor lysis syndrome (TLS) due to increased cell turnover as a complication of effective chemotherapy and radiotherapy, which lead to fast cell destruction. As a result of increased renal excretion, hyperuricemia can be responsible for acute renal insufficiency. Conger and Falk [1] reported a reduction of the glomerular filtration rate (GFR) due to tubular and vascular obstruction by urate deposition.

Andreoli [2] measured the urine excretion of urate, xanthine, and hypoxanthine from 19 children with acute lymphoblastic leukemia, who were being treated with allopurinol during tumor lysis. In the alkaline urine of these patients the urate and hypoxanthine excretions did not exceed maximal solubility, whereas xanthine did in 16 of 19 patients. In urine sediments from 8 patients, xanthine precipitates were found. These results indicate that acute renal insufficiency cannot always be explained by hyperuricemia and that high xanthine levels might have an effect on renal insufficiency.

Another mechanism might explain the acute renal insufficiency in TLS. In contrast to its action in relaxing vascular smooth muscle, adenosine produces renal vasocontraction [3]. The GFR is lowered by adenosine because the afferent arteriole is contracted while the efferent arteriole is somewhat relaxed. Adenosine can be formed by increased ATP catabolism during tumor cell destruction while patients are on chemotherapy. Leukemic cells contain a high ATP content [4]. These observations suggest that adenosine is at least partly responsible for renal insufficiency. However, half-lives of 0.6 s for adenosine were measured in blood [5]. Therefore, a high and continuous release of adenosine is needed during tumor lysis to affect renal function.

In conclusion, the mechanism which explains acute renal insufficiency is still unclear. More information could be obtained when plasma oxypurines and adenosine are measured during tumor lysis.

References

1. Conger JD, Falk SA (1977) Intrarenal dynamics in the pathogenesis and prevention of acute urate nephropathy. J Clin Invest 59: 786–793
2. Andreoli SP, Clark JH, McGuire WA, Bernstein JM (1986) Purine excretion during tumor lysis in children with acute lymphocytic leukemia receiving allopurinol: relationship to renal failure. J Pediatr 2: 292–298

3. Spielman WS, Arend LJ and Forrest Jr JN (1987) The renal and epithelial Actions of Adenosine. In: Gerlach E and Becker BF (eds) Topics and perspectives in adenosine research, Springer-Verlag, Berlin Heidelberg, p 249–260
4. De Abreu RA, van Baal JM, Bakkeren JAJM, de Bruyn CHMM, Schretlen EDAM (1982) A high performance liquid chromatographic assay for identification and quantification of nucleotides in lymphocytes and malignant lymphoblasts. J Chromatogr Biomed Appl 227: 45–54
5. Möser GH, Schrader J, Deussen A (1989) Turnover of adenosine in plasma of human and dog blood. Am J Physiol 256: C799–C806

J. G. PUIG

It would be interesting to know what the uric acid to creatine ratio in the Japanese paper was. I would like to emphasize that an increased urinary uric acid concentration may serve as a nidus for calcium oxalate precipitation, and that hyperuricosuria is a risk factor for calcium urolithiasis. This is not always preventable by purine-rich food restriction. We have shown that some patients with calcium oxalate stone disease are hyperuricosuric and that their increased urinary uric acid concentrations were due to a tubular defect causing urate wasting. In some of these patients we documented hypouricemia and the curious thing is that we treated these patients with allopurinol, even if they had hypouricemia.

Hypouricemia associated with cancer is well known and the only case I am aware of in which a uricosuric substance was found was medullary carcinoma of the thyroid. . . and the substance was calcitonin.

Hypouricemia has been well demonstrated to be associated with SIADA; this could serve for differential diagnosis with other hyponatremic conditions.

R. W. E. WATTS

Are you satisfied that the rising part of your curve for [14C] urate cumulative excretion against time is in fact more rapid in the hypouricemic patient than in the controls? It seems to me that they are not sufficiently different for us to be sure.

F. ROCH-RAMEL

How is urate transported by the proximal tubule of human kidneys? As mentioned by Dr. Sperling, in humans, as in other mammals urate undergoes bidirectional transport in the proximal tubule. Depending on the species, either net reabsorption or net secretion is observed. Man is a urate reabsorber. Many studies have been performed in vivo and in vitro in different mammals in order to investigate which mechanisms are involved in urate transport (Roch-Ramel and Weiner 1980; Kahn and Weinmann 1985). The most recent investigations concern studies on luminal (brush-border) and basolateral membranes isolated from proximal tubules of urate reabsorbers (mongrel dogs and rats) and urate secreters (pigs and rabbits). Data on transport at the basolateral membrane are still scarce, and further investigations are needed before understanding how urate is transported at this membrane. In contrast there are extensive data from brush-border membranes. It was demonstrated that in urate reabsorbtion urate is transported by urate-anion exchange, this mechanism being absent in urate secreters (Werner et al. 1980). Recently we obtained renal tissue from one patient undergoing nephrectomy for renal malignancy and we prepared brush-border membrane vesicles from tumor-free cortex. In these membranes, we could demonstrate the presence of a urate exchange mechanism. Thus, as in dogs and rats, there was urate exchange with chloride and hydroxyl ions. Preliminary data showed that pyrazinoate, but not *p*-aminohippurate, could inhibit the urate-chloride exchange. In humans, thus, the affinity of the urate exchanger mechanism for different organic anions differs from that of dogs and rats. In these two species both *p*-aminohippurate and pyrazinoate have affinity for the urate-anion exchanger.

Kahn AM, Weinman EJ (1985) Urate transport in the proximal tubule: in vivo and vesicles studies. Am J Physiol 249: F789–F798
Roch-Ramel F, Weiner IM (1980) Renal excretion of urate: factors determining the action of drugs. Kidney Int 18: 665–676
Werner D, Martinez F, Roch-Ramel F (1990) Urate and *p*-aminohippurate transport in the brush border membrane of the pig kidney. J Pharmacol Exp Ther 252: 792–799

W. Löffler

With cases of hereditary renal hypouricemia reported in the literature, description of results of pharmacological tests only fit the suggested classifications of this syndrome in a few patients, while in the majority it did not. Evaluation of results always have implied – though unspokenly – secretion of urate and drugs occurring at identical sites in tubule, but we cannot even be sure about this important prerequisite. My impression is that the question of whether secretion is normal cannot be answered in vivo by use of drugs, but only by giving a urate load. In these pharmacological studies we observe response or non-response to the drugs administered. I wonder if this isn't a better tool for classifying different defects in renal hypouricemia than calculating amounts of secretion and reabsorption.

As to clinical consequences of renal hypouricemia. I would like to add a third one. We gave allopurinol to a patient with renal hypouricemia due to drug-induced tubular toxicity and to one with the isolated hereditary defect of urate reabsorption. In both patients, renal excretion of oxipurinol was normal, while plasma levels of oxipurinol as well as excretion of hypoxanthine and xanthine were too low for the dose administered, thus demonstrating impaired response to the drug due to exaggerated oxipurinol clearance [1]. It would appear that renal hypouricemia, be it primary or secondary, is a biochemical marker of a renal drug wasting syndrome in humans. I would be interested in knowing whether hypouricemia treatment with theophylline, azethioprine, thioguanine or other purine drugs would affect the excretion of these drugs (or of metabolites) too.

Löffler et al. (1989) Klin Wochenschr 67: 47

6

Epidemiology of Hyperuricaemia

U. GRESSER and B. GATHOF

The importance of the clinical consequences of hyperuricaemia in man depends firstly on the *intensity* of clinical impairment and secondly on its *prevalence*.

It is well-known that a relationship exists between uric acid levels and the standard of living. In times with terrible conditions when people were poor, hyperuricaemia was a rare disorder. In days of prosperity, the consumption of purine-rich food and alcohol increased, and hyperuricaemia became more frequent.

Since the early 1960s, the standard of living in industrialised countries has improved, and thus the number of people with high uric acid levels has risen. For that reason we decided to investigate once more the serum uric acid levels in Bavaria, altogether the fourth study in our laboratory since 1962.

In autumn 1989 we examined uric acid levels in a group of 3200 blood donors and compared the results with 3 older studies from 1962 to 1984, using similar analytical methods in a comparable group of blood donors.

Figure 1 shows the distribution of serum uric acid levels in 2097 male and 1103 female blood donors examined in Southern Germany in 1989. In the women the mean uric acid level was 4.16 ± 0.96 mg/dl; in the men it was

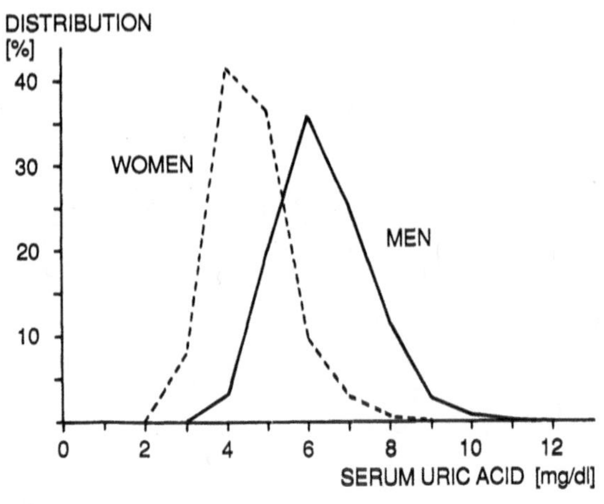

Fig. 1. Distribution of serum uric acid levels in 2097 male and 1103 female blood donors in Bavaria in 1989 (Gresser et al. 1990)

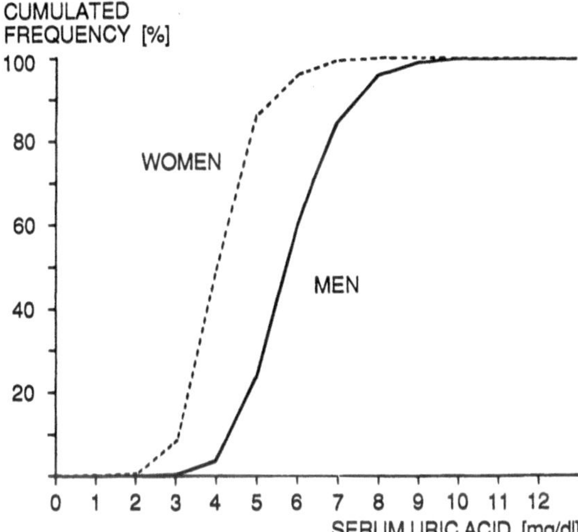

Fig. 2. Cumulated frequencies of serum uric acid levels in 2097 male and 1103 female blood donors in Bavaria in 1989 (Gresser et al. 1990)

5.90 ± 1.16 mg/dl. The difference between men and women was statistically significant. In Fig. 2, the results are shown as cumulated frequencies. There is a marked difference between women and men.

Figure 3 shows serum uric acid levels in relation to different age groups in the blood donors, giving the mean values, standard deviation and standard deviation of the means. Uric acid levels in women aged 18–20 years were significantly higher than in the group aged 21–30 years. The levels in women between 51 and 60 years of age were significantly higher than in women between 41 and 50 years of age. In men, the uric acid levels did not vary significantly among the different age groups.

Table 1 displays the results in relation to blood groups, with mean and standard deviation. Uric acid levels did not differ significantly with respect to blood groups in either men or women.

Table 1. Serum uric acid levels in blood donors from Bavaria in relation to blood groups, 1989. Values are given as mean $\pm$ standard deviation (Gresser et al. 1990)

Blood group (number of blood donors)	Serum uric acid levels (mg/dl)		
	Total	Women	Men
0 (1456)	5.31 ± 1.41	4.17 ± 1.02	5.91 ± 1.20
A (1231)	5.30 ± 1.34	4.19 ± 0.92	5.89 ± 1.14
B (357)	5.24 ± 1.36	4.08 ± 0.90	5.87 ± 1.13
AB (156)	5.31 ± 1.29	4.15 ± 0.73	5.96 ± 1.07

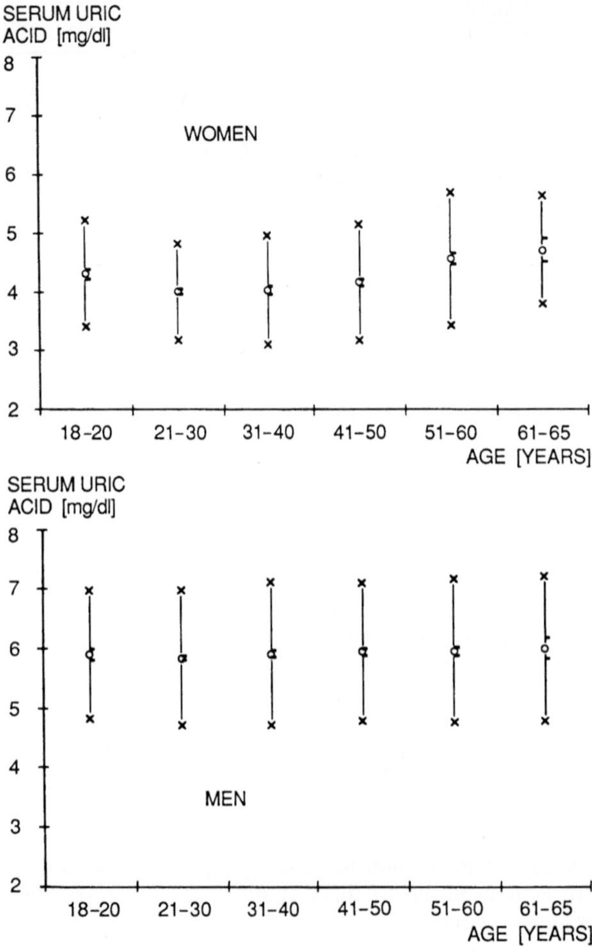

Fig. 3. Relation of serum uric acid levels to different age groups in 1103 female and 2097 male blood donors in 1989 (0 = mean, x = standard deviation, – = standard deviation of the mean) (Gresser et al. 1990)

Table 2 shows the serum uric acid levels in blood donors from different regions of Bavaria, also given as mean and standard deviation. Comparison of the results showed no significant difference in female blood donors, but men from Regensburg and the Bavarian Forest showed higher values than donors from the Munich or Augsburg areas. These findings may possibly be explained by a higher consumption of purines, especially beer, for which these areas are well-known.

Table 2. Serum uric acid levels in blood donors from different regions of Bavaria, 1989. Values are given as mean ± standard deviation (Gresser et al. 1990)

Region (number of blood donors)	Serum uric acid levels (mg/dl)		
	Total	Women	Men
Regensburg/Bavarian forest (419)	5.36 ± 1.37	4.19 ± 0.93	6.06 ± 1.09
Munich/Oberbayern (1103)	5.23 ± 1.37	4.11 ± 0.93	5.84 ± 1.17
Augsburg/Schwaben (1678)	5.34 ± 1.37	4.20 ± 0.98	5.90 ± 1.17

Table 3. Serum uric acid levels in Bavarian blood donors in 1962, 1971, 1984 and 1989. All studies were carried out by the same group. Values are given as mean ± standard deviation (Gresser et al. 1990)

Reference, year of study	Serum uric acid levels (mg/dl)	
	Men (n)	Women (n)
Zöllner (1968) 1962	4.86 ± 1.32 (265)	4.05 ± 1.29 (119)
Griebsch and Zöllner (1973) 1971	6.00 ± 1.22 (662)	4.35 ± 1.06 (337)
Löffler et al. (1989) 1984	5.60 (739)	4.10 (337)
Gresser et al. (1990) 1989	5.90 ± 1.16 (2097)	4.16 ± 0.96 (1103)

In Table 3, the mean values of uric acid levels between 1962 and 1989 are given. All studies were carried out by our research group on Bavarian blood donors. Uric acid levels were always determined enzymatically. Between 1962 and 1989 they rose by 0.11 mg/dl to 4.16 mg/dl in women and by 1.01 mg/dl to 5.90 mg/dl in men. In both men and women, the highest uric acid levels were measured in 1971. Those obtained in 1984 were intermediate between the 1971 and present values.

In Fig. 4, the cumulated frequencies of uric acid levels in female blood donors in 1962, 1971 and 1989 are compared. In women, there is almost no difference between the three studies. Contrary to this, in men there is an obvious increase in between 1962 and 1971. From 1971 to 1989 the values remained constant.

The risk of developing gout or certain renal disorders is related to the level of uric acid (Table 4). In our study (Tables 5, 6) 2.6% of the female and 28.6% of the male blood donors had uric acid values higher than 6.4 mg/dl and must therefore be considered hyperuricaemic.

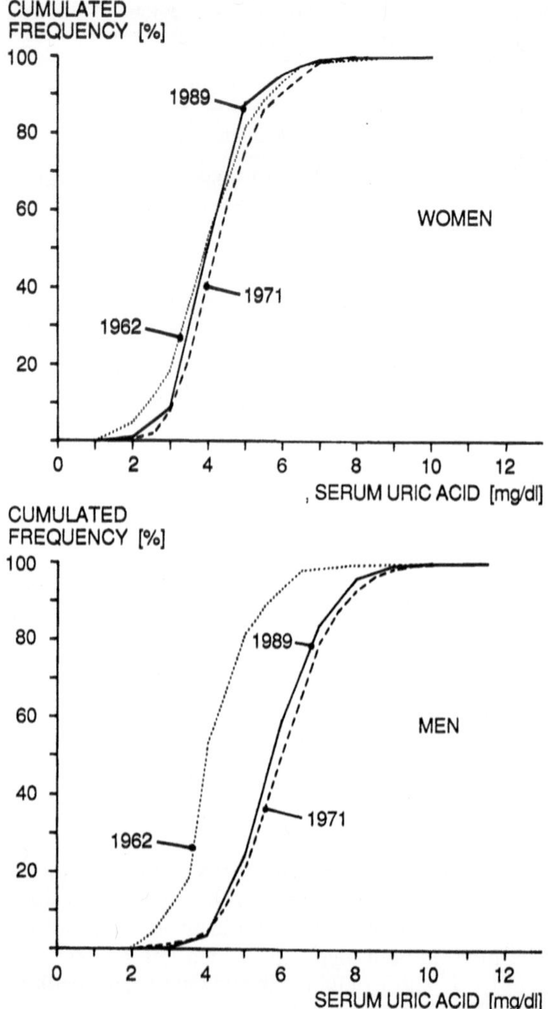

Fig. 4. Cumulated frequencies of uric acid levels in female and male blood donors in Bavaria in 1962, 1971 and 1989. (Data for this figure were extracted from Zöllner 1963 and Griebsch and Zöllner 1973)

Table 4. Relationship between uric acid levels and gouty arthritis

Reference	Serum uric acid levels (mg/dl)	Frequency of gouty arthritis
		Incidence
Hall et al.	>7	20.8
1967	>8	34.6
Campion et al.	7.0–7.9	2.0
1987	8.0–8.9	4.1
	9.0–9.9	19.8
	>10	30.5
		Prevalence
Zalokar et al.	6.0–6.9	2.3
1972	7.0–7.9	4.7
	8.0–8.9	11.4
	9.0–9.9	31.6
	>10	47.6
Isomaeki	>7	13.8
1969	>9	66.6

Table 5. Serum uric acid levels in male and female blood donors from Bavaria in 1989 (Gresser et al. 1990)

Uric acid (mg/dl)	Men		Women	
	(*n*)	%	(*n*)	%
≤1.0	0	0.0	1	0.1
1.1– 2.0	0	0.0	2	0.2
2.1– 3.0	6	0.3	88	8.0
3.1– 4.0	69	3.3	455	41.2
4.1– 5.0	419	20.0	399	36.2
5.1– 6.0	750	35.8	109	9.8
6.1– 7.0	530	25.3	35	3.2
7.1– 8.0	241	11.5	10	0.9
8.1– 9.0	62	2.9	2	0.2
9.1–10.0	16	0.8	1	0.1
10.1–11.0	1	0.0	0	0.0
11.1–12.0	1	0.0	1	0.1
12.1–13.0	0	0.0	0	0.0
≥13.1	2	0.1	0	0.0
Total	2097	100.0	1103	100.0

Table 6. Cumulated frequencies of serum uric acid levels in 2097 male and 1103 female blood donors in Bavaria, 1989 (Gresser et al. 1990)

Limit (mg/dl)	Men (%)	Women (%)
$\geq$ 6.1	40.7	4.4
$\geq$ 6.5	28.6	2.6
$\geq$ 7.1	15.4	1.3
$\geq$ 8.1	3.9	0.4
$\geq$ 9.1	1.0	0.2
$\geq$ 10.1	0.2	0.1
$\geq$ 11.1	0.1	0.1
$\geq$ 12.1	0.1	0.0
$\geq$ 13.1	0.1	0.0

Table 7. Prevalence of hyperuricaemia in different populations. *Question marks* indicate figures not contained in the respective publication. In the column „uric acid levels", fields were left blank when the information was not given in the publication. In Samoa different populations with different uric acid levels were examined. In this table, *Year* means the year of uric acid determination (Gresser et al. 1990)

Country Year, reference	Prevalence of hyperuricaemia (%)							
	>6.0 ♂	♀	$\geq$ 6.5 ♂	♀	>7.0 ♂	♀	>8.0 ♂	♀
West Germany								
1962 Zöllner (1963)			8.0	4.0				
1971 Griebsch and Zöllner (1973)	48.4	9.0	32.2	5.9	20.3	3.6	7.2	0.0
1989 Gresser et al. (1990)	40.7	4.4	28.6	2.6	15.4	1.3	3.9	0.4
East Germany								
1969 Thiele (1980)		1.8				2.4		
1978 Schröder (1982)		19.7				29.0		
Switzerland								
197? Bräuer et al. (1986)	34.4	20.0	28.8	10.1	19.2	9.3	6.7	3.8
France								
1965–1967 Zalokar et al. (1972)	43.2		28.4		17.6		5.4	
USA								
196? Hall et al. (1967)	22.0	3.3			4.8	0.5	1.0	0.0
1978–1980 Glynn et al. (1983)							11.3	
Canada								
1970–197? Munan et al. (1976)	44.0	14.2	26.3	6.6	16.9	3.3	6.3	1.2
Guayana								
1972 Bois et al. (1972)		40.7				22.8		
Samoa								
1978 Jackson et al. (1981)		23.3–29.5				36.4–43.3		

Table 8. Prevalence of hypouricaemia in different populations

Reference populations	(n)	Prevalence	Limit of uric acid (mg/dl)
Hisatome et al. 1989 Patients in general practice	3258	0.40	<2.0
Ramsdell and Kelley 1973 Hospital patients	6629	0.72	<2.0
Van Peenen 1973 Patients in general practice	5000	0.97	<2.0
Peretz et al. 1983 Hospital patients	2200	1.05 4.00	<2.0 <2.5

In Table 7, the prevalences of hyperuricaemia in different populations are compared. The first three lines show the Munich studies. The interesting fact is that since the upper limit for uric acid is 6.4 mg/dl, the percentage of hyperuricaemic people is *similar in different populations* between the years 1965 and 1989. Some 26.3%–32.2% of men and 2.6%–10.1% of women were found to be hyperuricaemic.

Only a few studies provide data on the prevalence of *hypouricaemia*. The limiting value is 2.0 mg/dl, and the prevalence of hypouricaemia was determined by various authors to be in the range of 0.4%–1.05% (Table 8). In our study (Table 5) 3 women of 3200 blood donors were found to be hypouricaemic (frequency 0.3% of the female blood donors).

For adjustment of our results, we collected some epidemiological data from Europe, Scandinavia, North and South America, some Pacific countries, the Near East and Africa. As in southern Germany, in the former East Germany (Table 9) uric acid levels have increased. Thiele and Schröder examined blood donors between 1969 and 1977. They found a constant rise in uric acid levels in men and women.

In the 1970s and 1980s in Switzerland, France and the UK (Table 10) uric acid levels of 5.3 to 6.1 mg/dl in men and 4.5 to 4.8 mg/dl in women were recorded. These values are near to those found in Germany.

Similar results were seen in Scandinavia (Table 11).

In the USA (Table 12) a large number of epidemiological studies on uric acid were carried out. As in Europe, the uric acid values in men increased from about 5 mg/dl in the 1950s to more than 6 mg/dl in the 1970s.

Healey et al. did an interesting study with people from the Philippines (Table 13). They compared the uric acid values of Philippinos living in the Philippines and those living in Hawaii or Seattle. The former had lower uric acid levels than those living in Hawaii or Seattle, who consumed more

Table 9. Uric acid levels in Germany. Values are given as mean ± standard deviation. *Figures in parentheses* indicate the number of subjects studied. *Question marks* indicate figures not found in the respective publication. In this table, *Year* means the year of uric acid determination (Gresser et al. 1990)

Country Year, reference	Population	Uric acid levels (mg/dl)	
		Men	Women
West Germany			
1962 Zöllner (1963)	Blood donors	4.86 ± 1.32 (265)	4.05 ± 1.29 (119)
1969 Haug et al. (1972)	Hospital patients	6.02 ± 1.38 (5656)	4.62 ± 1.18 (5248)
1971 Griebsch and Zöllner (1973)	Blood donors	6.00 ± 1.22 (662)	4.35 ± 1.06 (337)
1984 Löffler et al. (1989)	Blood donors	5.60 ± ? (739)	4.10 ± ? (337)
East Germany			
1969 Thiele and Schröder (1980)	Blood donors	4.2 ± ? (495)	3.4 ± ? (550)
1971	Blood donors	4.8 ± ? (566)	3.7 ± ? (633)
1973	Blood donors	5.5 ± ? (375)	4.4 ± ? (337)
1977	Blood donors	6.2 ± ? (687)	4.6 ± ? (313)
1980 Thiele and Schröder (1982)	Blood donors	6.3 ± ? (?)	5.2 ± ? (?)
198? Schröder et al. (1985)	Children (4 – 10 years)	5.0 ± 0.8 (40)	5.3 ± 0.9 (35)
	Children (10 – 16 years)	5.4 ± 0.8 (47)	5.0 ± 0.9 (81)
	Adults	5.5 ± 0.9 (294)	4.8 ± 1.1 (328)

Table 10. Uric acid levels in Europe. Values are given as mean $\pm$ standard deviation. *Figures in parentheses* indicate the number of subjects studied. *Question marks* indicate figures not found in the respective publication. In this table, *Year* means the year of uric acid determination (Gresser et al. 1990)

Country Year, reference	Population	Uric acid levels (mg/dl)	
		Men	Women
Switzerland 197? Bräuer et al. (1976)	Patients in general practice	5.6 ± ? (104)	4.5 ± ? (317)
France 1965 – 1967 Zalokar et al. (1972)	Male employees	5.88 ± 1.19 (23.923)	–
197? Bonaiti et al. (1976)	Population Rodome	5.36 ± 1.12 (113)	4.50 ± 0.94 (229)
	Population Camurac	6.14 ± 1.26 (69)	4.80 ± 1.15 (127)
UK 1978 – 1980 Cook et al. (1986)	Male patients in general practice	5.9 ± 1.15 (7.730)	–

Table 11. Uric acid levels in Scandinavia. Values are given as mean $\pm$ standard deviation. *Figures in parentheses* indicate the number of subjects studied. *Question marks* indicate figures not found in the respective publication. In this table, *Year* means the year of uric acid determination (Gresser et al. 1990)

Country Year, reference	Population	Uric acid levels (mg/dl)	
		Men	Women
Norway 197? – 197? Helgeland et al. (1978)	Male patients with hypertension	5.5 ± ? (150) 6.0 ± ?	before and after 3 years thiazide therapy
		5.7 ± ? (150) 5.3 ± ?	Control group before and after 3 years
Sweden 1968 – 1969 Bengtsson and Tibblin (1974)	Female population		3.6 – 4.4 ± 1.1 – 1.5 (1462)
Finland 196? Isomaeki (1969)	Country population	5.0 ± 1.1 (737)	4.0 ± 1.2 (1048)
	City population	5.2 ± 1.2 (90)	4.4 ± 1.2 (90)

Table 12. Uric acid levels in North and South America. Values are given as mean ± standard deviation. *Figures in parentheses* indicate the number of subjects studied. *Question marks* indicate figures not found in the respective publication. In this table, *Year* means the year of uric acid determination (Gresser et al. 1990)

| Country | Population | Uric acid levels (mg/dl) | |
Year, reference		Men	Women
USA			
195?–? Hall et al. (1967)	Population Framingham	5.12±1.11 (2062)	4.0±0.94 (2489)
1956–1960 Mikkelsen and Dodge (1965)	Population Tecumseh	4.94±? (1663)	4.18±? (1725)
1962–1965		5.25±? (1663)	4.36±? (1725)
196? Dunn et al. (1963)	Employees	4.77±1.13 (532)	–
	Clerks	5.73±1.21 (339)	–
1969–1972 Kasl and Sandler (1977)	Cadets West Point	5.17±0.78 (1130)	–
1961–1963 Glynn et al. (1983)	Male population Boston	5.77±0.87 (1141)	–
1975–1978		6.53±1.15 (1141)	–
1975–1979 Stewart et al. (1979)	Patiens older than 65 years	6.30±1.3 (490)	5.38±? (829)
Canada			
1970–197? Munan et al. (1976)	Population Sherbrooke	5.80±1.32 (558)	4.74±1.10 (663)
Guayana			
197? Bois and Feingold (1972)	3 tribes	6.2±1.3 (22)	5.6±1.3 (18)

purine-rich food. Healey et al. concluded that ethnic origin is less relevant than standard of living regarding the development of hyperuricaemia.

The uric acid levels in men measured in Israel (Table 14) in the 1960s are comparable with those in the Munich study of 1962.

To conclude, our study is in good agreement with publications from other industrialised countries. During the 1950s and 1960s an increase in uric acid

Table 13. Uric acid levels in some Pacific countries. Values are given as mean ± standard deviation. *Figures in parentheses* indicate the number of subjects studied. *Question marks* indicate figures not found in the respective publication. In this table, *Year* means the year of uric acid determination (Gresser et al. 1990)

Country Year, reference	Population	Uric acid levels (mg/dl)	
		Men	Women
Hawaii 1965–1969 Yano et al. (1977)	Men of Japanese origin	5.99 ± 1.51 (7971)	–
Philippines 196? Healey et al. (1967)	Philippinos in – Philippines – Hawaii – Seattle	 5.2 ± 1.3 (483) 6.1 ± 1.3 (60) 6.3 ± 1.4 (113)	 – – –
Japan 1973–1974 Okada et al. (1980)	Population Hisayama	5.31 ± 1.08 (861)	4.74 ± 1.10 (1147)
Australia 196? Jeremy and Towson (1971)	Male employees. clerks	6.28 ± 1.23 (500)	–
New Zealand 198? Gibson et al. (1984)	Maori men – normouricaemic – asymptomatic with hyperuricaemia – with gout	 6.3 ± 0.75 (79) 8.0 ± 0.5 (26) 8.66 ± 1.6 (10)	 – – –
Micronesia 1968–1969 Reed et al. (1972)	Different populations	6.2–7.1 ± 1.3–1.5 (778)	4.9–5.4 ± 1.2–1.4 (946)
Samoa 1978 Jackson et al. (1981)	Country population	6.87 ± 1.18 (356)	5.46 ± 1.13 (319)
	City population	6.72 ± 1.43 (384)	5.27 ± 1.23 (415)

levels was observed. Since the early 1970s, this increase has levelled out, and in the past 15–20 years uric acid levels have remained constant. In Bavaria at the end of the 1980s 2.6% of the female blood donors and 28.6% per cent of the male blood donors were hyperuricaemic and thus had an increased risk of gout, nephrolithiasis, nephropathy and other clinical disorders.

Table 14. Uric acid levels in the Near East and Africa. Values are given as mean ± standard deviation. *Figures in parentheses* indicate the number of subjects studied. *Question marks* indicate figures not found in the respective publication. In this table, *Year* means the year of uric acid determination (Gresser et al. 1990)

Country Year, reference	Population	Uric acid levels (mg/dl)	
		Men	Women
Israel 1963 Herman and Goldbourt (1982)	Male clerks over 40 years old	4.75 ± ? (8627)	–
1965	Male clerks over 40 years old	5.18 ± ? (8237)	–
1968	Male clerks over 40 years old	5.25 ± ? (8051)	–
Sudan 197? Ibrahim (1975)	Patients	3.8 ± 1.1 (400)	? (100)

References

Bengtsson C and Tibblin E (1974) Serum uric acid levels in women. Acta Med Scand 196: 93–102

Bois E et Feingold J (1972) Génétique de l'uricémie: étude de trois tribus amérindiennes de la Haute-Guyane Française. Ann Génét 15: 257–264

Bonaiti C, Constans J et Valdiguié P (1976) Etude génétique et épidémiologique de l'uricémie dans une population pyrénéenne. Rev Epidem et Santé Publ 24: 469–478

Bräuer R, Clémencon G and Otto C (1976) Serumharnsäurewerte im Patientengut der Allgemeinpraxis. Schweiz Rundschau Med 65: 1094–1098

Campion EW, Glynn RJ and DeLabry LO (1987) Asymptomatic hyperuricemia. Risks and consequences in the normative aging study. Am J Med 82: 421–426

Cook DG, Shaper AG, Thelle DS and Whitehead TP (1986) Serum uric acid, serum glucose and diabetes: relationships in a population study. Postgrad Med 62: 1001–1006

Dodge HJ (1970) Observations on the distribution of serum uric acid levels in participants of the Tecumseh, Michigan, community health studies. J Chron Dis 23: 161–172

Dunn JP, Brooks GW, Mausner J, Rodnan GP and Cobb S (1963) Social class gradient of serum uric acid levels in males. JAMA 185: 431–436

Gibson T, Waterworth R, Hatfield P, Robinson G and Bremner K (1984) Hyperuricaemia, gout and kidney function in New Zealand Maori men. Br J Rheumatol 23: 276–282

Glynn RJ, Campion EW and Silbert JE (1983) Trends in serum uric acid levels 1961–1980. Arthr Rheum 26: 87–93

Gresser U, Gathof B, and Zöllner N (1990) Uric Acid Levels in Southern Germany 1989. A Comparison with Studies from 1962, 1971 and 1984. Klin Wochenschr 68: 1222–1228

Griebsch A und Zöllner N (1973) Normalwerte der Plasmaharnsäure in Süddeutschland – Vergleich mit Bestimmungen vor 10 Jahren. Z Klin Chem 11: 348–356

Hall AP, Barry PE, Dawber TR and McNamara PM (1967) Epidemiology of gout and hyperuricemia. A long-term population study. Am J Med 42: 27–37

Haug H, Spahn U, Hermann G and Gathof G (1972) Harnsäure. Alter, Geschlecht und sozialer Status. Eine Untersuchung an 10904 Patienten der Medizinischen Universitäts-Poliklinik Würzburg. Med Welt 23: 1321–1325

Healey LA (1975) Epidemiology of hyperuricemia. Arthr Rheum 18: 709–712

Healey LA, Skeith MD, Decker JL and Bayani-Sioson PS (1967) Hyperuricemia in Filipinos: Interaction of heredity and environment. Am J Hum Gen 19: 81–85

Helgeland A, Hjermann I, Holme I and Leren P (1978) Serum triglycerides and serum uric acid in untreated and thiazidetreated patients with mild hypertension. Am J Med 64: 34–38

Herman JB and Goldbourt U (1982) Uric acid and diabetes: observations in a population study. Lancet 2: 240–243

Hisatome I, Ogino K, Kotake H, Isiko R, Saito M, Hasegawa J, Mashiba H and Nakamoto S (1989) Cause of persistent hypouricaemia in outpatients. Nephron 52: 13–16

Ibrahim SA (1975) Hyperuricaemia in Sudanese. J Trop Med Hyg 78: 47–48

Isomaeki H (1969) Hyperuricaemia in northern Finland. An epidemiological study of serum uric acid in rural, urban and hospital populations. Ann Clin Res Suppl 1: 1–62

Jackson L, Taylor R, Faaiuso S, Ainuu SP, Whitehouse S and Zimmet P (1981) Hyperuricaemia and gout in western Samoans. J Chron Dis 34: 65–75

Jeremy R and Towson J (1971) Serum urate levels and gout in Australian males. Med J Austr 1: 1116–1118

Kasl S and Sandler D (1977) An epidemiologic study of serum cholesterol and serum uric acid in a population of healthy young men. Milit Med 853–857

Löffler W, Hartmann D, Hogh-Binder A, Schreiber E, Schewe S (1989) Trends in serum uric acid levels in Southern Germany, 1961–1984. Ann Nutr Metab 33: 219–220

Mikkelsen WM, Dodge HJ and Valkenburg H (1965) The distribution of serum uric acid values in a population unselected as to gout or hyperuricemia. Tecumseh, Michigan 1959–1960. Am J Med 39: 242–251

Munan L, Kelly A and Petitclerc C (1976) Population serum urate levels and their correlates. The Sherbrooke regional study. Am J Epidemiol 103: 369–382

Okada M, Takeshida M, Ueda K, Omae T and Hirota Y (1980) Factors influencing the serum uric acid level. A study based on a population survey in Hisayama town, Kyushu, Japan. J Chron Dis 33: 607–612

Van Peenen HJ (1973) Causes of hypouricemia. Ann Int Med 78: 977–978

Peretz A, Decaux G and Famaey JP (1983) Hypouricemia and intravenous infusions. J Rheum 10: 66–70

Ramsdell CM and Kelley WN (1973) The clinical significance of hypouricaemia. Ann Intern Med 78: 1312–1314

Reed D, Labarthe D and Stallones R (1972) Epidemiologic studies of serum uric acid levels among Micronesians. Arthr Rheum 15: 381–390

Schröder HE, Mank H, Mende T, Heinrich JJ (1985) Verhalten des Serumsäurespiegels von Kindern im Vergleich zu Erwachsenen sowie Häufigkeit von Purinstoffwechselstörungen und Begleitkrankheiten bei Kindern aus gichtbelasteten Familien. Z Ges Inn Med 40: 221–226

Stewart RB, Yost RL, Hale WE and Marks RG (1979) Epidemiology of hyperuricemia in an ambulatory elderly population. J Am Geriatr Soc 27: 552–554

Thiele P und Schröder HE (1980) Epidemiologie und Klinik der Hyperurikämie und Gicht. Z Ärztl Fortbild 74: 655–658

Thiele P und Schröder HE (1982) Epidemiologie der Hyperurikämie und Gicht. Z Ges Inn Med 37: 406–410

Yano K, Rhoads GG and Kagan A (1977) Epidemiology of serum uric acid among 8.000 Japanese-American men in Hawaii. J Chron Dis 30: 171–184

Zalokar J, Lellouch J, Claude JR and Kuntz D (1972) Serum uric acid in 23.923 men and gout in a subsample of 4.257 men in France. J Chron Dis 25: 305–312

Zöllner N (1963) Eine einfache Modifikation der enzymatischen Harnsäurebestimmung – Normalwerte in der deutschen Bevölkerung. Z Klin Chem 1: 178–182

Pathogenesis of Monosodium Urate Crystal-Induced Inflammation

R. TERKELTAUB

Introduction

Acute articular and periarticular inflammation and chronic articular destructive changes are well-recognized consequences of the deposition, in articular and periarticular tissues, of crystals of the monosodium salt of uric acid (MSU). MSU crystals directly or indirectly activate a remarkable number of humoral and cellular inflammatory mediator systems, and this is reflected in the clinical features of a typical acute gouty paroxysm, i.e., acute onset, severe pain, edema and erythema extending beyond the joint margin, neutrophil influx and activation, and systemic manifestations. In this chapter, our current understanding of the pathogenesis of MSU-crystal-associated inflammation is reviewed.

Humoral Mediators in Gout

MSU crystals activate the classic complement pathway in vitro (reviewed in Terkeltaub et al. 1989) and can bind and induce the cleavage of macromolecular C1 in the absence of immunoglobulin (Giclas et al. 1979). However, classic pathway activation is amplified by IgG and C-reactive protein. Alternative pathway activation occurs in vitro under conditions under which the classic pathway activation is selectively inhibited (Doherty et al. 1983). In addition, direct cleavage of C5 to C5a and C5b can occur via a stable C5 convertase formed on the crystal surface. MSU crystals also activate Hageman factor and the contact system of coagulation in vitro (reviewed in Terkeltaub et al. 1989), leading to the generation of kallikrein, bradykinin, plasmin, and other inflammatory mediators (Ginsberg et al. 1980).

The physiologic significance of these findings is supported by evidence of complement activation in a substantial proportion of gouty synovial fluids and the detection of kinins in joint fluids in both spontaneous and experimental MSU-crystal-induced inflammation. However, neither complement nor contact coagulation system activation appears essential for gouty arthritis to occur in experimental models, and acute gout has been reported in humans with Hageman factor deficiency. Such observations reinforce the inherent redundancy of host inflammatory responses to MSU crystals.

Cell-Derived Mediators in Gout

The central roles of neutrophil influx and neutrophil activation are supported by the striking accumulation of these cells in both the joint fluid and synovial membrane in acute gout, where they phagocytose crystals actively and aggregate and degranulate in the microvasculature in areas remote from crystals (Agudelo and Schumacher 1973). Second, experimental urate crystal-induced synovitis is diminished in neutrophil-depleted animals (Phelps and McCarty 1966). Third, a number of agents that suppress neutrophil function are effective in preventing and terminating acute gouty inflammation (discussed below).

Neutrophils exposed to MSU crystals release lysosomal proteases, superoxide, and lipoxygenase-derived products of arachidonic acid, including leukotriene B4 (LTB4) (Serhan et al. 1984). A chemotactic, 15 kD. protein (Bhatt and Spilberg 1988) termed crystal-induced chemotactic factor (CCF) (Spilberg and Mandell 1982) also appears to be transcriptionally activated and secreted in neutrophils after phagocytosis of MSU and certain other particulates. Importantly, CCF has an amino acid composition distinct from that of IL-8 (Baggiolini et al. 1989), which is also transcribed by activated neutrophils (Streiter et al. 1990) CCF causes neutrophil infiltration and synovitis in vivo, and LTB4 and a molecule resembling CCF have been identified in human acute gouty synovial fluids.

Cells other than neutrophils also appear to be involved in the pathogenesis of gouty inflammation. Urate crystals are known to stimulate fibroblasts in vitro, and the crystals interact physically with synovial lining cells and mononuclear phagocytes on gouty joints. Furthermore, acute gout has been described in the absence of neutrophils in human synovial fluid. Importantly, MSU crystals stimulate the release of vasoactive prostaglandins, proteases, and a number of proinflammatory cytokines [including IL-1, tumor necrosis factor (TNF)-α, IL-6, and IL-8] (Di Giovine et al. 1987; Guerne et al. 1989) from cultured monocytes and synoviocytes.

The participation of synovial mast cells, platelets, or both in acute gout is theoretically possible; platelets are among the earliest cells to mediate inflammatory responses, and their interaction with urate crystals in vitro is well-recognized (Jaques and Ginsberg 1982). Mast cells are recognized to reside in synovia, and stimulation of these cells in vitro by C3a, C5a, and IL-I results in the release of a variety of inflammatory mediators, including histamine. In this regard, early articular swelling has been diminished by antihistamines in experimental MSU-crystal-induced inflammation.

Basic Mechanisms of MSU-Crystal-Induced Cellular Activation

MSU crystals induce perturbation and delayed lysis of plasma membranes and model liposomes. In addition, rapid responses not mediated by membrane lysis are prominent, including platelet serotonin secretion and neutrophil superoxide anion and lysosomal protease secretion (reviewed in Terkeltaub et al. 1989). Interestingly, membranes and liposomes not bearing cholesterol are not lysed by MSU crystals.

The negatively charged oxygen atoms prominent on the MSU crystal surface impart a net negative surface charge. However, atomic components with a partial positive charge are also exposed on the crystal surface (Mandel 1976). Thus, MSU crystals are believed to associate with plasma membranes by (a) hydrogen bonding, with crystals acting as hydrogen acceptors in interactions with positively charged phospholipid polar head groups and as hydrogen donors in interactions with membrane glycoproteins and (b) formation of electrostatic bonds with polar membrane structures. Consistent with this hypothesis is the evidence that MSU crystals interact with both positively and negatively charged electron spin resonance membrane probes (Herring et al. 1986).

Phagocytosis of urate crystals by neutrophils is followed by rapid dissolution of the phagolysosomal membrane. This process has been termed "suicide sac formation" because the internal release of lysosomal contents supervenes, followed by cellular swelling and death. However, cell death following phagocytosis of membranolytic crystals may also depend on an influx of extracellular calcium into the damaged cell.

The mechanisms whereby MSU crystals induce functional leukocyte responses are heterogeneous. Opsonization of the crystals is clearly unnecessary, although crystal-bound IgG enhances the capacity of MSU to stimulate a number of cells. MSU crystals appear to activate membrane G proteins (including Gi α2) in neutrophils (Terkeltaub et al. 1990b). Though MSU crystals can increase membrane permeability through lytic effects (Weissmann and Rita 1972), they also induce rapid cytosolic calcium mobilization, modulated by phosphatidylinositol-4,5-bisphosphate (PIP2) hydrolysis and inositol-1,4,5-trisphosphate generation in neutrophils (Onello et al. 1990). However, unlike neutrophil activation induced by chemotactic factors, MSU-crystal-induced PIP2 hydrolysis, cytosolic calcium mobilization, and functional responses do not require the activation of a pertussis-toxin-sensitive G protein (Terkeltaub et al. 1990b).

PIP2 hydrolysis is not the sole indication of membrane phospholipase activation by MSU. For example, MSU crystals also induce direct phospholipase A2 activation and release of a phospholipase-A2-activating protein in leukocytes (Bomalaski et al. 1990).

MSU-crystal-induced leukocyte membrane activation events are likely modulated by both membrane perturbation and the considerable reactivity of the surface of the MSU crystal, which gives it the ability to bind and potentially crosslink and cluster membrane proteins, including adhesion molecules. For example, in platelets, the membrane integrin Gp IIb/IIIa clearly binds to urate crystals, and it modulates urate-induced platelet serotonin secretion (Jaques and Ginsberg 1982). Crosslinking and clustering of freely mobile membrane proteins by multivalent ligands such as MSU crystals may be analogous to the effect on leukocytes of crosslinking of certain membrane proteins (including Fc receptors, Kimberly et al. 1990; Krutmann et al. 1990) and solid-phase bound CD44 and CD45 (Webb et al. 1990), which can result in pertussis-toxin-insensitive cytosolic calcium mobilization (Kimberly et al. 1990) or cytokine induction.

Initiation, Propagation, and Termination of Acute Gout
(Figure 1)

MSU crystals liberated from synovial microtophi or precipitated de novo are believed to activate the described humoral and cellular mediator cascades. Early vasodilation, enhanced vascular permeability, and pain in gouty arthritis are likely mediated by vasoactive prostaglandins, kinins (which also potentiate prostaglandin synthesis via release of membrane arachidonate), complement peptides, and histamine. Pain signals may theoretically mediate acute gout via the release from nociceptive afferent sensory nerve fibers of substance P, which has a number of proinflammatory functions (Lotz et al. 1987).

Although neutrophils appear to be the usual effector arm of acute gouty inflammation, they are virtually absent in normal joint fluid. Thus, humoral and resident cell-derived mediators [including LTB4 and platelet activating factor (PAF)] probably trigger neutrophil ingress into joints (Figure 1) MSU-crystal-induced release of IL-1 and TNF-α from monocytes and synovial lining cells could promote neutrophil ingress via the induction of adhesion protein expression by the endothelial cells of postcapillary venules. IL-1 and TNF-α are also known to induce the release of the neutrophil chemotactic/activating cytokine IL-8 from mononuclear phagocytes, fibroblasts, and a number of other cells (Baggiolini et al. 1989). In this regard, IL-8 appears to be the major neutrophil chemotactic factor released from monocytes activated by MSU crystals in vitro, and it is abundant in acute gouty joint fluids (Terkeltaub et al. 1990c).

The release of neutrophil-derived mediators (e. g., CCF, LTB4, lysosomal proteases) in response to contact with both intraarticular MSU crystals and fluid-phase mediators (e. g., LTB4, C5a, kallikrein, TNF-α, IL-8) is believed to establish a cycle of further neutrophil ingress, neutrophil activation, and amplification of inflammation.

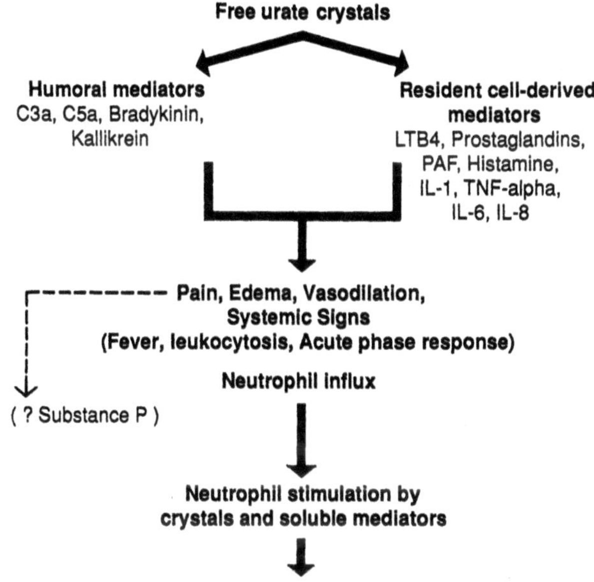

Fig. 1. Hypothetical mechanisms involved in initiation and propagation of acute gouty arthritis

Systemic signs (including low grade fever, leukocytosis, and the hepatic acute phase protein response) often accompany local manifestations in acute gouty inflammation. These appear to be consequences of the capacity of MSU crystals to directly (and indirectly) induce IL-1, TNF-α, IL-8, and IL-6 release from activated mononuclear phagocytes and synovial lining cells.

The self-limitation characteristic of acute gouty inflammation has been remarked upon since the time of Hippocrates. Factors other than MSU crystal dissolution or sequestration must play a role in terminating attacks, as free MSU crystals are often found in synovial fluid for many weeks after the subsidence of an acute gouty paroxysm. The following factors could contribute:

–(a) Tachyphylaxis to mediators (Colditz and Movat 1984), e. g., stimulus-specific desensitization of neutrophils to chemotactic factors and inhibition of neutrophil phagocytosis of MSU by CCF (Spilberg and Mandell 1982); (b) the limited (days) normal functional lifespan of neutrophils (Savill et al 1989). Both of these factors may make continued recruitment of new neutrophils to the gouty inflammatory locus necessary for prolonging acute inflammation (Haslett et al. 1989).

– Inactivation and clearance of mediators (e. g., omega-oxidation of LTB4 and inactivation of bradykinin, C3a and C5a by carboxypeptidases).

– Shedding of soluble Fc and TNF-α receptors by activated neutrophils (Huizinga et al. 1990; Porteau and Nathan 1990).

– Induction and release from cells of molecules that exert antiinflammatory effects (reviewed in Arend and Dayer 1990); e. g., PGE$_2$, which inhibits neutrophil function; the recently characterized IL-1 receptor level antagonist protein (Hannum et al. 1990); TGF-β (Transforming growth factor-beta) (which inhibits IL-1 receptor expression); and IL-6, which can inhibit TNF-α release under certain conditions (Aderka et al. 1989) and can, along with IL-1, induce central adrenocortitotropic hormone (ACTH) release with subsequent endogenous adrenal glucocorticoid release.

– Changes in the adsorbed proteins during the evolution of the gouty paroxysm (e. g., binding of neutrophil lysosomal enzymes to MSU crystals can displace IgG from the crystal surface and render them less able to stimulate neutrophils in vitro (Rosen et al. 1986). Other mechanisms whereby molecules absorbed to MSU crystals surfaces might determine the crystal's inflammatory potential are discussed below.

Variable Inflammatory Potential of MSU Crystals: Effects of Absorbed Proteins

No direct correlation exists between the amount of MSU crystal deposition and the severity of acute gout (reviewed in Terkeltaub et al. 1989). For example, large amounts of MSU crystals ("joint milk") may be aspirated from joints that show little or no sign of inflammation. In other patients, few crystals are detected despite severe acute gouty synovitis. A striking absence of inflammation about subcutaneous deposits of MSU crystals in the rule, and some patients with chronic tophaceous gout give no history of acute attacks. A multitude of factors, including host responsiveness, the inhibitory effects of glycosaminoglycans (GAGs) on leukocyte responsiveness to MSU crystals and neutrophil chemotaxis, and variable crystal morphology and surface structure (Perl-Treves and Addadi 1988) could account for these observations.

Much attention has focused on the possibility that proteins adsorbed to MSU crystal surfaces could be the critical determinant of their inflammatory potential. Although opsonization with isolated IgG enhances the intrinsic capacity of MSU crystals to stimulate leukocytes, crystals incubated with whole serum are markedly less stimulatory for leukocytes. The effects of serum are due to apo-B-bearing lipoproteins (Terkeltaub et al. 1984). Low density lipoprotein (LDL), the predominant apo B lipoprotein, suppresses cellular responses to MSU by binding to the crystal surface, thereby physically inhibiting particle-cell interaction and phagocytosis (Terkeltaub et al. 1986a, b). Apo B is both necessary and sufficient for this activity of LDL.

Importantly, MSU crystals in quiescent tophaceous synovial deposits are physically associated with variable amounts of surface proteins and lipids (Agudelo and Schumacher 1973), and removal of this coating appears to enhance greatly their ability to activate leukocytes (Gordon and Roberts-Thompson 1986). The lipids in tophi include cholesteryl esters, which are predominantly carried by plasma LDL. Furthermore, LDL binds to MSU crystals in vivo, particularly in the later stages of acute gout (Ortiz-Bravo et al. 1990). In addition, apo E can be bound to MSU crystals in vivo (Terkeltaub et al. 1990a). Apo E has a number of functional properties in common with apo B, including the ability to bind MSU crystals and blunt their capacity to activate neutrophils. Importantly, apo E, unlike apo B, is synthesized within synovial joints by cells of the monocyte/macrophage lineage, and thus it exemplifies a locally produced factor capable of markedly altering the inflammatory potential of MSU crystals.

Basis for Therapeutic Strategies

Acute gouty inflammation is generally satisfactorily treated by colchicine, nonsteroidal antiinflammatory drugs (NSAIDs), or adequate doses of local or systemic glucocorticoids (reviewed in Terkeltaub et al. 1989). In addition, low doses of colchicine and NSAIDs are effective in prophylaxis. Colchicine therapy is most effective in acute gout when administered in the earliest stages of the attack. It inhibits many neutrophil functions, including certain responses to LTB4, CCF, and IL-8. It also suppresses degranulation and MSU-crystal-induced LTB4 and CCF release from neutrophils. However, it does not appear to diminish crystal-induced cytokine release from monocytes. NSAIDs are probably effective via inhibition of neutrophil functions, suppression of pain and increased vascular permeability via inhibition of prostaglandin generation, and other factors. The therapeutic efficacy of glucocorticoids may occur in large part via suppression of proinflammatory cytokine transcription, of neutrophil activation, and via the induction of lipocortins (Camussi et al. 1990).

MSU crystal deposition is associated not only with episodic acute inflammation but also with chronic synovitis, articular erosions, and cartilage and subchondral osseous destruction. Because the MSU-crystal-induced release from resident mononuclear phagocytes and synovial lining cells of cytokines and proteases likely fuels chronic inflammation and connective tissue degradation, adequate and expeditious measures to reduce hyperuricemia and to promote resorption of crystals are imperative. In this regard, articular destructive changes and deformities can progress despite uric-acid-lowering therapy that adequately diminishes further episodes of acute gout (McCarthy et al.

1990). Thus, guidelines for the therapeutic target level of serum uric acid and strategies for monitoring tophi may need to be individualized.

Finally, because of the precise chemical definition of the physical agonist, further study of the mechanisms of MSU-crystal-associated synovitis also represents an exquisite opportunity to understand better the mechanisms capable of regulating inflammation.

References

Aderka D, Le J, Vilcek J (1989) IL-6 inhibits lipopolysaccharide-induced tumor necrosis factor production in cultured human monocytes, U937 cells, and in mice. J Immunol 143: 3517–3523

Agudelo C, Schumacher HR (1973) The synovitis of acute gouty arthritis. A light and electron microscopic study. Hum Pathol 4: 265–269

Arend WP, Dayer J-M (1990) Cytokines and cytokine inhibitors or antagonists in rheumatoid arthritis. Arthritis Rheum 33: 305–315

Baggiolini M, Walz A, Kunkel SL (1989) Neutrophil-activating peptide-1/interleukin-8, a novel cytokine that activates neutrophils. J Clin Invest 84: 1045–1049

Bhatt A, Spilberg I (1988) Purification of crystal induced chemotactic factor from human neutrophils. Clinical Biochem 21: 341–345

Bomalaski JS, Baker DG, Brophy LM, Clark MA (1990) Monosodium urate crystals stimulate phospholipase A2 enzyme activities and the synthesis of a phospholipase A2-activating protein. J Immunol (In press)

Camussi G, Tetta C, Bussolino F, Baglioni C (1990) Antiinflammatory peptides (antiinflammins) inhibit synthesis of platelet-activating factor, neutrophil aggregation, and chemotaxis, and intradermal inflammatory reactions. J Exp Med 171: 913–927

Colditz, IG, Movat HZ (1984) Desensitization of acute inflammatory lesions to chemotaxins and endotoxin. J Immunol 133: 2163–2168

Di Giovine FS, Malawista SE, Nuki G, Duff GW (1987) Interleukin-1 (IL-1) as amediator of crystal arthritis: stimulation of T cell and synovoal fibroblast mitogenesis by urate crystal-induced IL-1. J Immunol 138: 3213–3218

Doherty M, Whicher JT, Dieppe PA (1983) Activation of the alternative pathway complement by monosodium urate monohydrate crystals and other inflammatory particles. Ann Rheum Dis 42: 285–291

Giclas PC, Ginsberg MH, and Cooper NR (1979) Immunoglobulin G independent activation of the classical complement pathway by monosodium urate crystals. J Clin Invest 63: 759–765

Ginsberg MH, Jaques B, Cochrane CG, Griffin JH (1980) Urate crystal-dependent cleavage of Hageman factor in human plasma and synovial fluid. J Lab Clin Med 95: 497–506

Gordon TP, Roberts-Thompson PJ (1986). Preliminary evidence for the presence of an inhibitor on the surface of natural monosodium urate crystals. Arthritis Rheum 29: 1172–1173

Guerne PA, Terkeltaub R, Zuraw B, Lotz M (1989) Stimulation of IL-6 production in human monocytes and synoviocytes by inflammatory microcrystals. Arthritis Rheum 32: 1443–1452

Hannum CH, Wilcox CJ, Arend WP, Joslin FG, Dripps DJ, Heimdal PL, Armes LG, Sommer A, Eisenberg SP, Thompson RC (1990) Interleukin-1 receptor antagonist activity of a human interleukin-1 inhibitor. Nature 343: 336–340

Haslett, C, Jose PJ, Giclas PC, Williams TJ, Henson PM (1989) Cessation of neutrophil influx in C5a-induced acute experimental arthritis is associated with loss of chemoattractant activity from the joint space. J Immunol 142: 3510–3517

Herring FG, Lam E, Burt HM (1986) A spin label study of the membranolytic effects of crystalline monosodium urate monohydrate. J Rheumatol 13: 623–630

Huizinga TWJ, de Haas M, Kleijer M, Nuijens JH, Roos D, von den Borne AEG (1990) Soluble Fc gamma Receptor III in human plasma originates from release by neutrophils. J Clin Invest 86: 416–423

Krutmann J, Kirnbauer R, Kock A, Schwarz T, Schopf E, May LT, Sehgal PB, Luger TA (1990) Cross-linking Fc receptors on monocytes triggers IL-6 production. Role in anti-CD3-induced T cell activation. J Immunol 145: 1337–1342

Jaques BC, Ginsberg MH (1982) The role of cell surface proteins in platelet stimulation by monosodium urate crystals. Arthritis Rheum 25: 508–521

Kimberly RP, Ahlstrom JW, Click ME, Edberg JC (1990) The glycosyl phosphatidylinositol-linked FcgammaRIII$_{PMN}$ mediates transmembrane signalling events distinct from FcgammaRII. J Exp Med 171: 1239–1255

Lotz, Carson D, Vaughan J (1987) Substance P activation of rheumatoid synoviocytes: Neural pathway in pathogenesis of arthritis. Science 235: 893–895

Mandel NS (1976) The structural basis of crystal-induced membranolysis. Arthritis Rheum 19: 439–455

McCarthy GM, Barthelemy CR, Veum JA, and Wortmann RL (1990) Influence of antihyperuricemic therapy on the clinical and radiographic progression of gout. Arthritis Rheum 33: S54 (abstract)

Onello E, Traynor-Kaplan A, Sklar L, Terkeltaub R (1991) Mechanism of neutrophil activation by an unopsonited inflammatory particulate. Arthritis Rheum, in press

Ortiz-Bravo E, Clayburne G, Sieck M, Rothfuss S, Schumacher HR (1990) Immunolabeling of proteins coating monosodium urate(MSU) crystals in sequential samples from acute gouty arthritis and MSU induced inflammation in the rat subcutaneous air pouch. Arthritis Rheum 33: S55 (abstract)

Perl-Treves D, Addadi L (1988) A structural approach to pathological crystallizations. Gout: the possible role of albumin in sodium urate crystallization. Proc R Soc Lond 235: 145–159

Phelps P and McCarty DJ (1966) Crystal-induced inflammation in canine joints. II. Importance of polymorphonuclear leukocytes. J Exp Med 124(1): 150

Porteau F, Nathan C (1990) Shedding of tumor necrosis factor receptors by activated human neutrophils. J Exp Med 172: 599–607

Rosen MS, Baker DG, Schumacher HR, Cherian PV (1986) Products of polymorphonuclear cell injury inhibit IgG enhancement of monosodium urate-induced superoxide production. Arthritis Rheum 29: 1473–1479

Savill JS, Wyllie AH, Henson JE, Walport MJ, Henson PM, and Haslett C (1989) Macrophage phagocytosis of aging neutrophils in inflammation. Programmed cell death in the neutrophil leads to its recognition by macrophages. J Clin Invest 83: 865–875

Serhan CN, Lundberg U, Weissmann G Samuelsson B (1984) Formation of leukotrienes and hydroxy acids by human neutrophils and platelets exposed to monosodium urate. Prostaglandins 17: 563–581

Spilberg I, Mandell B (1982) Crystal-induced chemotactic factor. In: Weissmann G (ed) Advances in Inflammation Research, vol 5. Raven Press, New York, pp 57–65

Streiter RM, Chensue SW, Standiford TJ, Basha MA, Showell HJ, Kunkel SL (1990) Disparate gene expression of chemotactic cytokines by human mononuclear phagocytes. Biochem Biophys Res Comm 166: 886–891

Terkeltaub R, Curtiss LK, Tenner AJ, Ginsberg MH (1984) Lipoproteins containing apolipoprotein B are a major regulator of neutrophil responses to monosodium urate crystals. J Clin Invest 73: 1719–1725

Terkeltaub R, Dyer C, Martin J, Curtiss LK (1990a) Apolipoprotein E (apo E) inhibits the capacity of monosodium urate crystals to stimulate neutrophils: Characterization of intraarticular apo E and demonstration of apo E binding to urate crystals in vivo. J Clin Invest (In press)

Terkeltaub R, Ginsberg M, McCarty DJ (1989) Pathogenesis and treatment of crystal-induced inflammation. In: McCarty DJ (ed) Arthritis and Allied Conditions. Lea and Febiger, Philadelphia, pp 1691–1710

Terkeltaub R, Martin J, Curtiss LK, Ginsberg M (1986a) Apolipoprotein B mediates the capacity of low density lipoprotein to suppress neutrophil stimulation of particulates. J Biol Chem 261: 15 662–15 667

Terkeltaub R, Sklar LA, Mueller H (1990b) Neutrophil activation by inflammatory microcrystals of monosodium urate monohydrate utilizes pertussis toxin-insensitive and sensitive pathways. J Immunol 144: 2719–2724

Terkeltaub R, Smeltzer D, Curtiss L, Ginsberg M (1986b) Low density lipoprotein inhibits the physical interaction of phlogistic crystals and inflammatory cells. Arthritis and Rheumatism 29: 363–369

Terkeltaub R, Zachariae C, Santoro D, Martin J, Peveri P, Matsushima K (1991) Monocyte-derived neutrophil chemotactic factor/IL-8 is a potential mediator of crystal-induced inflammation. Arthritis Rheum, in press

Webb DSA, Shimizu Y, Gizs AA, Seventer V, Shaw S, Gerrard TL (1990) LFA-3, CD44, and CD45: Physiologic triggers of human monocyte TNF and IL-1 release. Science 249: 1295–1297

Weissmann G, Rita GA (1972) Molecular basis of gouty inflammation: Interaction of monosodium urate crystals with lysosomes and liposomes. Nature [New Biol] 240: 167–172

Crystal-Associated Inflammation: Some Mechanisms of Cellular Activation

G. Nuki

Acute inflammation in association with crystals of monosodium urate is thought to be mediated by the presence of polymorphonuclear leucocytes (PMN) both in acute gouty arthritis and in experimentally induced crystal arthritis. Support for this hypothesis includes the massive accumulation of PMN in inflamed synovium and synovial fluid, the striking diminution of experimentally induced urate crystal synovitis following neutrophil depletion by cytotoxic drugs [1] or PMN-specific anti-serum [2] and the clinical effect of colchicine, a drug which inhibits many PMN functions [3]. Acute gouty arthritis can, however, occur in the absence of neutrophils [4], and some more recent studies have focussed on the potential role of monocytes [5, 6], resident macrophages, fibroblasts [7] and synoviocytes [8] as cells which could be responsible for the initial induction and chronic pathology in urate-crystal-mediated inflammation. Increasingly, evidence is pointing to a central role for soluble cytokines such as interleukin (IL)-1 [7], IL-6 [9], IL-8 [10] and tumour necrosis factor α (TNF-α) as mediators of urate-crystal-induced inflammation and tissue damage.

Crystals of monosodium urate (MSU) but not calcium pyrophosphate dihydrate (CPPD) or hydroxyapatite (HA) are dose-dependent stimulators of IL-1 [7] and TNF-α mRNA synthesis, protein production and release [11], although all three crystal types are potent stimulators of PMN superoxide anion production [12]. Cytokine stimulation and release by MSU crystals is independent of phagocytosis or adsorbed serum [6, 7, 11], and the time courses for production and release of IL-1 α and β and TNF-α differ greatly [11].

The presence of extra-cellular MSU crystals in the joints of patients between attacks of gouty arthritis [13], the absence of inflammatory reponse to crystals lodged in various connective tissue sites and the inconstant inflammatory response to experimental intra-articular injection of MSU crystals in human volunteers [14] all suggest that MSU crystals are necessary but not sufficient for the induction of acute gouty arthritis.

Further research on the role of soluble cytokines, soluble cytokine receptors and anti-cytokines in crystal-associated diseases may lead to new approaches to therapy as well as to a better understanding of the pathogenesis of these disorders.

References

1. Phelps P, McCarty DJ (1966) Crystal induced inflammation in canine joints II. Importance of polymorphonuclear leucocytes. J Exp Med 124: 150–166
2. Chang YH, Gralla EJ (1968) Supression of urate crystal induced canine joint inflammation by heterologous antipolymorphonuclear leucocyte serum. Arthritis Rheum 11: 145–150
3. Wallace SL (1974) Colchicine. Semin Arthritis Rheum 3: 369–381
4. Ortel RW, Newcombe DS (1974) Acute gouty arthritis and response to colchicine in the virtual absence of synovial fluid leucocytes. New Eng J Med 190: 363–364
5. Duff GW, Atkins E, Malawista SE (1983) The fever of gout: urate crystals activate endogenous pyrogen production from human and rabbit mononuclear phagocytes. Trans Assoc Am Physicians 96: 234–235
6. Malawista SE, Duff GW, Atkins E, Cheung HS, McCarty DJ (1984) Crystal induced endogenous pyrogen production. A further look at gouty inflammation. Arthritis Rheum 28: 1039–1043
7. Di Giovine FS, Malawista SE, Nuki G, Duff GW (1987) Interleukin 1 (IL-1) as a mediator of crystal arthritis: stimulation of T cell and synovial fibroblast mitogenesis by urate crystal induced IL-1. J Immunol 138: 3213–3218
8. Wigley FM, Fine IT, Newcombe DS (1983) The role of the human synovial fibroblast in monosodium urate crystal induced synovitis. J Rheumatol 10: 602–611
9. Houssiau FA, Devogelaer JP, Van Damme J, Nagant de, Deuxchaisnes C, Van Snick J (1988) Interleukin-6 in synovial fluid and serum of patients with rheumatoid arthritis and other inflammatory arthritides. Arthritis Rheum 31: 784–788
10. Terkeltaub R, Zacheriae C, Santoro D, Martin J, Peveri P, Matsushima N (1990) IL-8 as a potential medicator of crystal induced synovitis. Arthritis Rheum 33: (suppl) 320
11. Di Giovine FS (1988) The production of interleukin 1 and tumour necrosis factor by human monocytes and evidence for a role in arthritis. PhD Thesis University of Edinburgh
12. Palit J, Di Giovine FS, Dickens E, Duff GW, Nuki G (1986) Extracellular superoxide anion generation in response to pro-inflammatory crystals; selective stimulation of monocytes by monosodium urate. Brit J Rheumatol 25 (Supplement 1) 21
13. Gordon T, Bertouche J, Walsh B, Brooks P (1982) Monosodium urate crystals in asymptomatic joints. J Rheumatol 9: 967–969
14. Seegmiller JE, Howell RR, Malawista SE (1962) The inflammatory reaction to sodium urate: its possible relationship to the genesis of acute gouty arthritis. JAMA 180: 469–475

Questions and Comments Raised for Discussion

J. G. PUIG

Asymptomatic tophaceous gout is more common in women than in men, and I wonder whether there are intersexual differences with respect to humoral mediators and resident-cell humoral mediators?

G. VAN DEN BERGHE

What is the specificity of the effects observed with uric acid crystals on neutrophil activation? To what extent are they obtained with other crystals and to what extent does the steric structure of uric acid resemble that of other particulate stimuli, of neutrophils, for example, zymosan?

With respect to the self-limiting nature of the effects of urate crystals, has the possibility been looked into that the crystals might provoke a release of adenosine, which has been shown by B. Cronstein and his co-workers to inhibit neutrophil activation?

The Course of Chronic Gout with Special Reference to Extra-articular Manifestations and Joints Not Affected by Acute Attacks

J. T. SCOTT

The Tophus

The characteristic lesion of chronic gout is the tophus (Latin, rough porous stone), which consists of a multicentric deposit of fine needle-shaped crystals, often arranged radially, associated with an interstitial matrix and a surrounding foreign-body granuloma of epithelioid cells and giant cells, many of which are multinucleate (Fig. 1). The crystals are those of monosodium urate monohydrate: granular and amorphous urates are also present. With fresh deposition of urate the intervening inflammatory tissue tends to disappear, leaving large chalky or stony concretions.

The nature and significance of the matrix are uncertain. It has been shown to contain lipids and glycosaminoglycans which are presumably formed between the crystals as part of a tissue response, but such tissue alterations may themselves help to precipitate or maintain the development of the tophus (Sokoloff 1957). Urate deposition tends to occur in connective tissues rich in proteoglycans, particularly cartilage. The suggestion that proteoglycan aggregates of connective tissue are capable of initiating urate precipitation, losing this property on degradation, has not been confirmed (Perricone and Brandt 1978). With time the matrix may become partially calcified.

The course of chronic gout is naturally dependent upon the effectiveness of treatment and the degree to which the serum level of urate is controlled. Not all patients with gout proceed to develop tophi that are clinically obvious, and the pattern of evolution is variable. The extent of tophus formation is proportional to the duration of the disease and the height of the serum uric acid level (Gutman 1973). Yü (1974) showed how the prevalence of tophi fell progressively from 53% of patients in 1948–1953 to 17% in 1969–1973, doubtless owing to the influence of uricosuric treatment and later allopurinol. In a British study conducted in the late 1960s, Grahame and Scott (1970) found subcutaneous tophi in 75 of 354 patients (21%). By contrast, tophi were found in no fewer than 26 of 42 cases (62%) of secondary gout associated with myeloproliferative diseases, in which the serum urate level is higher than in primary gout (Yü 1965).

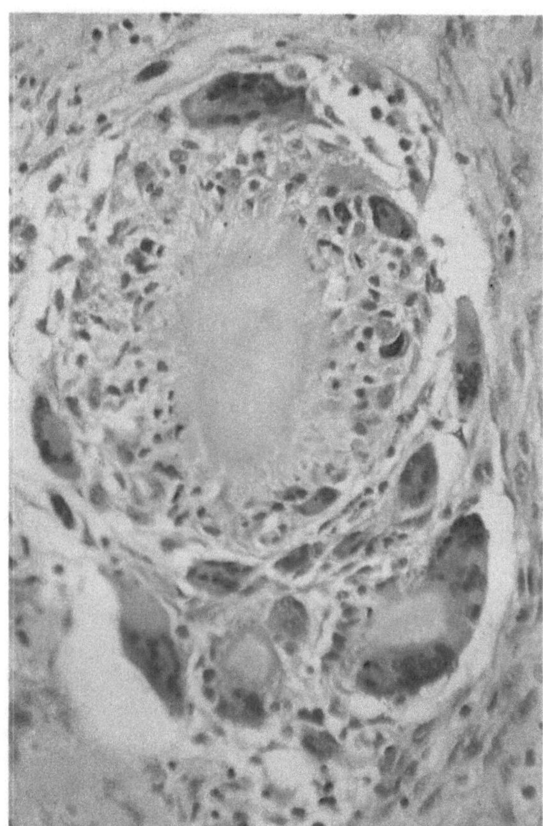

Fig. 1. Microphotograph ($\times$ 120) of periarticular gouty tophus showing oval area of matrix (from which crystals have been dissolved out) surrounded by foreign-body giant cells.

Sites of Tophus Formation

Deposits of urate are common in articular and other cartilage, synovial membrane, tendon sheaths, bursae, subcutaneous tissue and interstitial tissue of the kidneys, a subject which has been considered elsewhere.

In the joints themselves, the articular cartilage becomes coated with white chalky urate, and crystals are also formed within its superficial portions, as well as in synovial (Fig. 2), capsular and periarticular (Fig. 3) tissues. In the marrow of subchondral bone, tophus formation leads to collapse of the articular cartilage and "punched-out" lesions with their characteristic radiological appearance. Further progressive changes include disintegration of cartilage with secondary osteoarthritis and proliferation of marginal bone,

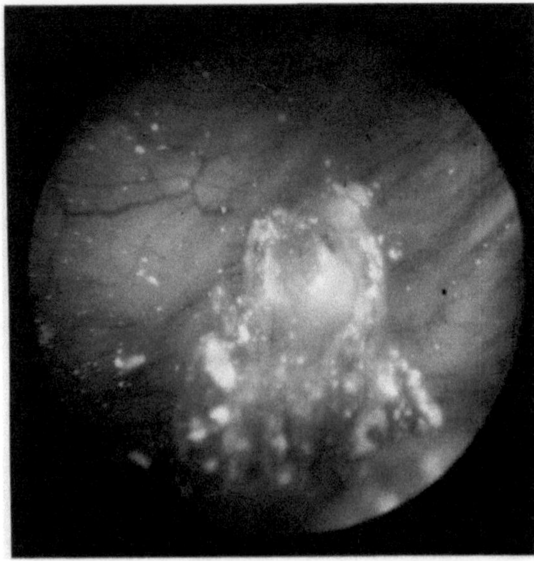

Fig. 2. Urate deposition on synovial membrane in the knee as seen through the arthroscope.

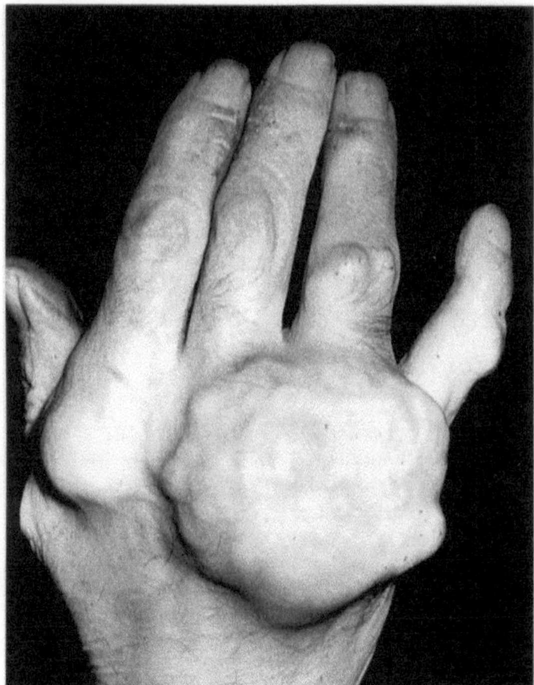

Fig. 3. Gross periarticular tophi in the hand.

obliteration of joint structure by urate deposition, proliferative tophaceous synovitis and occasionally fibrous or bony ankylosis.

Chronic joint changes usually follow repeated acute attacks but can develop insidiously in a previously unaffected joint. Acute attacks may continue to occur in the same joint but tend to cease late in the course of the disease. Such permanent changes are usually found in a number of different situations and are often prominent in the proximal and distal interphalangeal joints of the fingers, where periarticular tophi lead to bizarre, asymmetrical swelling. The skin overlying such tophi becomes thinned and shiny and through it can be seen the white mass of underlying sodium urate, which may later discharge itself as the skin breaks and ulcerates. Recurrent ulceration of this sort can be very troublesome, but infection is rarely a problem.

The distribution of chronic joint involvement is similar to that of acute gouty arthritis, with predominantly peripheral involvement, although deformity of the hands is more striking than in the feet (Fig. 4). Gouty arthritis in the wrists or flexor tendon sheaths occasionally causes a carpal tunnel syndrome (De Sèze and Phankim-Koupernik 1964; Champion 1969), and corresponding lesions in the lower limb have been reported to produce a tarsal tunnel syndrome (Edwards et al. 1969). Tophaceous deposits occur in association with olecranon, patellar and other bursae which become distended with fluid or thick, grumous, caseous material stuffed with urate crystals. The predilec-

Fig. 4. Chronic tophaceous deposits following trauma. The patient was a cricketer (wicket-keeper).

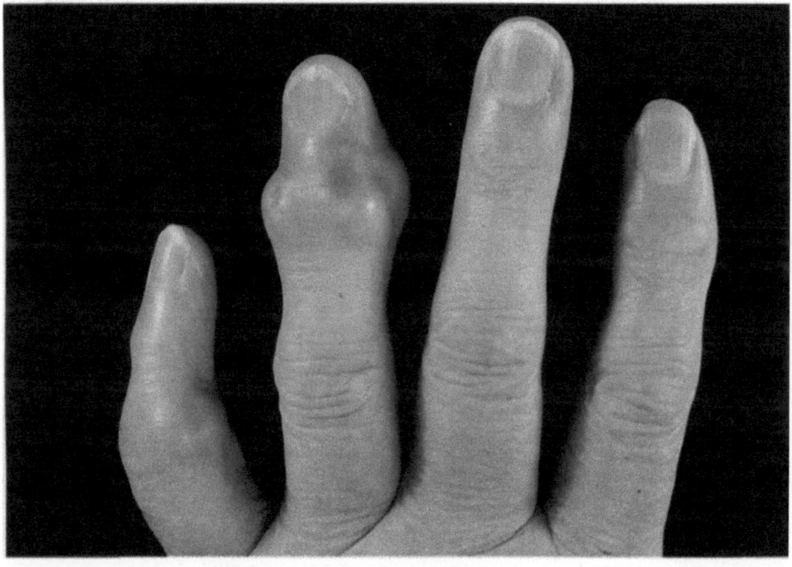

tion of urate deposition for cartilage is seen in non-articular structures, typically the helix of the ear, where tophi form small white excrescences usually about 1–4 mm in size, and the tarsal plates of the eyelids.

Of the 59 tophaceous patients reported by De Sèze et al. (1958), 36 had tophi in the ears, 32 in the hands, 27 in the feet, 24 over the elbows and 5 over the knees.

Subcutaneous tophi can occur well away from joints and are found, for

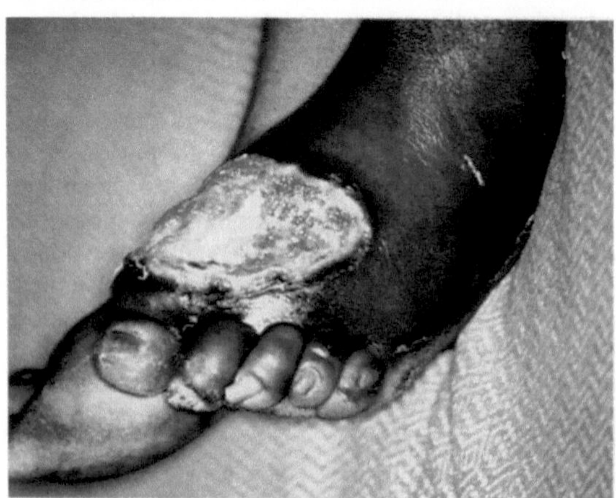

Fig. 5. Ulcerating tophus in the foot of a South African patient.

Fig. 6. Superficial collection of fluid tophaceous material.

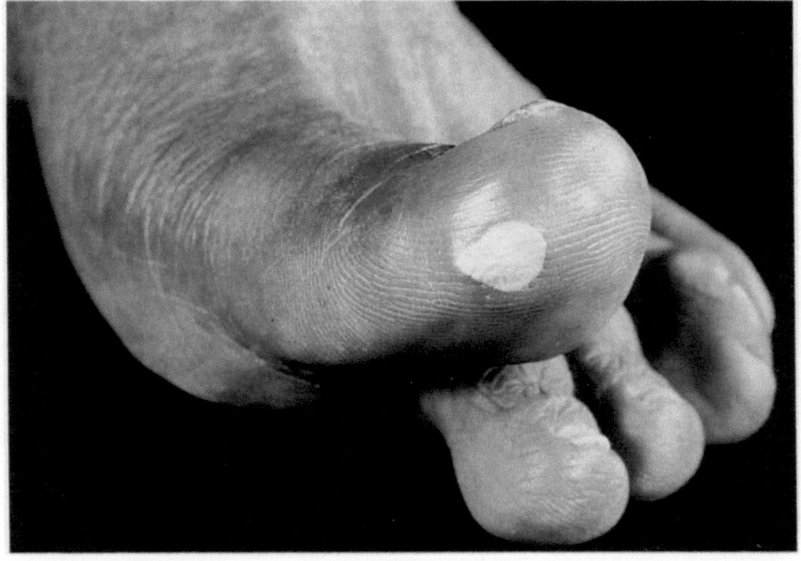

example, as abundant nodular deposits on the limbs and digits. They are painless and cause little trouble unless they ulcerate, discharging white chalky matter (Fig. 5). Subcutaneous deposition of urate can occasionally take the form of extensive superficial collections of white fluid resembling pus (Fig. 6).

Sites of tophaceous deposits are listed in Table 1. Some of these will be considered further.

Table 1. Sites of tophaceous deposits

Common	Rare	Never
Articular cartilage	Vertebrae and discs	Voluntary muscle
Other articular and periarticular		
structures	Heart	Liver
	Pericardium	Spleen
Cartilage elsewhere	Pleura	Lungs
Bursae	Larynx	Nervous tissue
Tendon sheaths	Intestine	
Subcutaneous tissue	Eyes	
Bone	Tongue	
Kidney	Bronchi	
	Meninges	
	Penis	

Bone

As already mentioned, deposits of urate are common in subchondral epiphyseal bone. Gout has also been implicated as an aetiological agent in osteonecrosis (aseptic necrosis) of the femoral head. Serre et al. (1963) studied hip radiographs in 150 patients with gout and found 3 with non-traumatic osteonecrosis of the femoral head. Examining the synovial membrane from the hip joint in 68 patients with idiopathic osteonecrosis, McCollum et al. (1968) demonstrated the presence of monosodium urate in 12, 8 of them with clinical gout and a further 3 with hyperuricaemia. Hunder et a. (1968) described a patient with gout and osteonecrosis in whom at surgery the femoral head and surrounding synovial membrane were found to be covered with urate crystals. The nature of this apparent association has not been elucidated. Is it conceivable that acute gout in the hip joint (a rare event) could increase intra-articular pressure to the extent that the blood supply is impaired or that the same effect could be produced by extensive bony deposition of urate? It seems unlikely. Alternatively, it is possible that urate could be deposited on already damaged cartilage and bone in a hyperuricaemic individual. Yet again, other factors may be operating, particularly excessive alcohol consumption, not uncommon among with patients gout and an aetio-

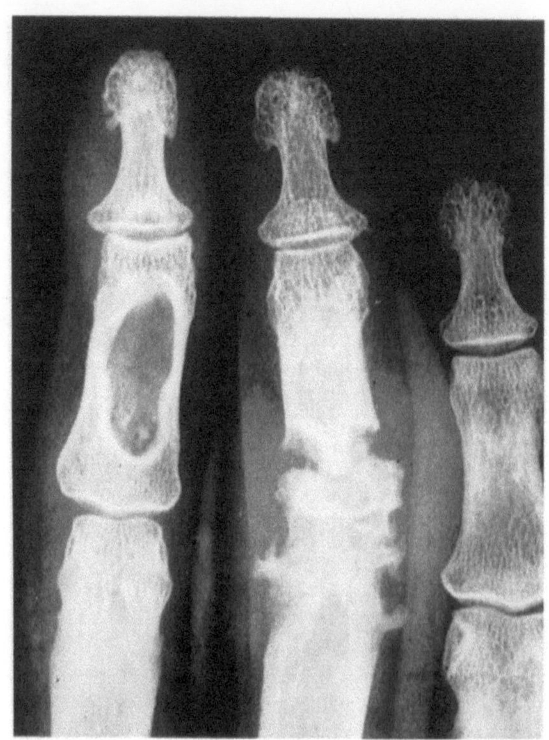

Fig. 7. Detail of hand X-radiograph of a patient with chronic tophaceous gouty arthritis. The proximal interphalangeal joint on the right shows the usual changes of bone destruction resulting from articular and para-articular tophaceous deposition. On the left a tophus has been formed in the shaft of the middle phalanx quite apart from neighbouring joints.

logical factor in some cases of osteonecrosis. Further careful clinico-pathological documentation is needed. The association does not appear to be common: no evidence of osteonecrosis was found with radiographs of the pelvis carried out in two large series of patients with gout (Rotes-Querol and Munoz Gomez 1965; Stockman et al. 1980).

Also of interest are tophaceous deposits which are laid down within the shafts of long bones, distant from any affected joint and with no soft-tissue tophi adjacent to the bone. They are occasionally seen in the phalanges (Fig. 7). Mahapatro et al. (1985) describe such a biopsied lesion within a clavicle.

The Axial Skeleton

Gout is a disorder involving the peripheral joints, but urate deposition can occur in the vertebrae, discs, spinal joints and approximating structures, especially if there is gross tophaceous disease elsewhere. It is only within the

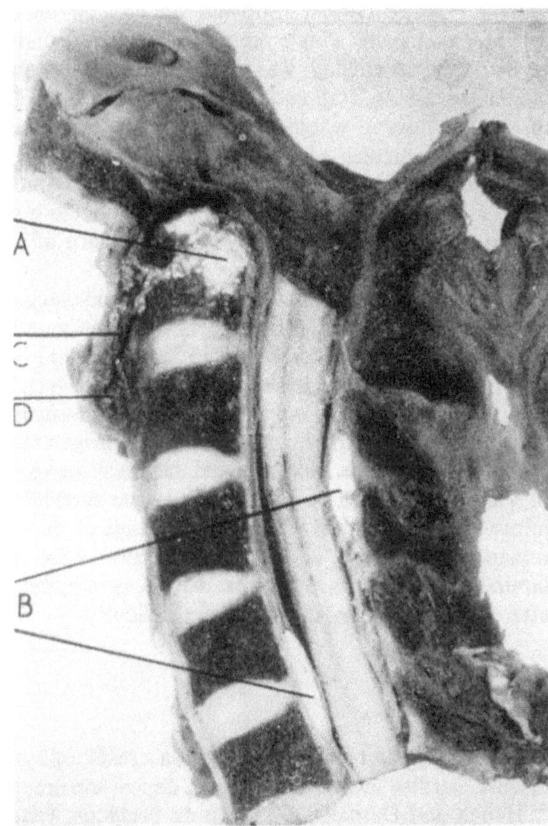

Fig. 8. Sagittal section through upper cervical vertebra, showing urate deposits in odontoid process of the axis (A); dura mater (B); subluxation of atlas vertebra (C); tophaceous material enclosed in fibrous sac D.
From Kersley *et al.* 1950, with kind permission of the authors and Editor, *Annals of the Rheumatic Diseases.*

cord itself that urate deposits do not occur. Such cases are rare, but there are several well-documented instances.

Kersley et al. (1950) described a patient with pain in the neck but with no neurological signs, in whom a band of tophaceous deposit lay between the base of the skull and the atlas, which had become eroded and fractured (Fig. 8). Vertebrodiscal lesions were described by Lichtenstein et al. (1956) and Vinstein and Cockerill (1972): in these studies the primary deposition of urate appeared to take place within the intervertebral discs with erosion of the adjacent bony end-plate. However, a careful autopsy study by Lagier and MacGee (1983) in an 84-year-old woman with polyarticular gout showed severe erosion of the second lumbar vertebral body due to urate deposition. Radiological signs had existed for many years. Comparison was made between a further small tophus and a Schmorl's node on two neighbouring thoracic vertebrae. The tophus had produced gradual destruction of the vertebral plate bone cortex, followed by erosion on the deep surface of the cartilaginous plate which otherwise appeared undamaged. The Schmorl's node, on the other hand, was associated with disc degeneration and vertebral plate remodelling. Hall and Selin (1960) described a patient with gout, dying of renal failure, in whom urate deposition was found in the capsules, ligaments and articular cartilage of the 4th and 5th lumbar and first sacral posterior articulations, with some in the discs. Gout involving the sacro-iliac joints – both acute and tophaceous – was noted by Malawista et al. (1965), who went on to discover radiological evidence of sacro-iliac disease in 7 of 95 patients with gout.

Extradural spinal deposition of urate can also occur at all levels, sometimes with dire neurological consequences such as quadriparesis (Sequeira et al. 1981), paraplegia (Koskoff et al. 1953; Litvak and Briney 1973) and paraplegia with cervical radiculopathy (Magid et al. 1981). The patient described by Wald et al. (1979) had only back pain with no neurological signs, but urate deposition in the extradural space had destroyed the pedicles of the 4th and 5th lumbar vertebrae and scalloped the posterior vertebral bodies. The patient of Varga et al. (1985), with extensive urate deposition in the pedicles, facetal joints and ligamentum flavum at the level of the 5th lumbar vertebra, was remarkable in that no peripheral tophi were present. Decompression laminectomy appears to have been successful in most of these cases, but only after a certain amount of diagnostic difficulty.

The Heart

Although the heart may be enlarged as a result of hypertensive cardiovascular disease, cardiac lesions due to urate deposition are extremely rare.

Hench and Darnall (1933), citing previous writers who agreed that true gouty endocarditis was very rare and gouty myocarditis practically non-existent, stated a case in which complete heart block was found to be caused by a large urate tophus affecting the conduction bundle. Virtanen and Halonen (1969) noted transient total heart block during an attack of gout.

Bunim and McEwen (1940) and Traut et al. (1954) described tophi in mitral leaflets. Pund et al. (1960) found a large tophus at the base of a mitral valve together with deposits of urate in valve leaflets and myocardium (in which tissue urate deposition must be very rare indeed). Scalapino et al. (1984) reported a man with chronic tophaceous gout and a previous history of rheumatic fever. At mitral valve replacement the leaflets were found to be thickened and fused by chronic rheumatic endocarditis with a superadded deposition of urate. The patient of Gawoski et al. (1985) was an old man with gout, renal stones, myocardial ischaemia and aortic incompetence. The aortic valve was replaced: its thickened and deformed cusps contained chalky white material consisting of massive deposits of crystalline and amorphous urate.

Other Organs

Tophaceous deposits are sometimes seen in the eyelid, but involvement of the globe itself is rare and difficult to evaluate because early reports ("the hot eye of gout") verge on the mythological. Some of them were reviewed by McWilliams (1952) who described a patient with confirmed conjunctival tophi. Corneal deposits of urate have been seen in band keratopathy (Fishman and Sunderman 1966), and Slansky and Kuwabara (1968) described a patient with a history of hyperuricaemia, acute gouty arthritis and nephrolithiasis in whom scintillating corneal crystals were seen on slit-lamp examination, epithelial scrapings showing the presence of crystals which were identified as urate. Frauenfelder et al. (1982) reported cataracts in association with allopurinol therapy. Liu et al. (1988) failed to confirm this but did discover an unusual morphological thinning of the anterior clear zone of the lens in patients taking the drug.

Tophi can occasionally involve the cartilage of the nasal septum and larynx, reports of which were reviewed by Lefkovits (1965), who himself noted a white spur extending beneath a vocal cord near the cricothyroid joint, which on excision was found to be a gouty tophus. A second nodule arose from a tracheal cartilage.

With the exception of the kidney, deposition of urate in the abdominal viscera is virtually unknown, although Hawkins et al. (1965) found tophi in the mucosa, submucosa and serosa of the small intestine. The kidneys were also involved, but no other viscera. Remarkably, the patient was the brother of the above-mentioned case of Kersley et al. (1950) with erosion of the atlas.

Muscle is one of the tissues in which tophi do not form, except by extension along fascial planes from the region of affected joints, but crystals of urate were found in muscle biopsy specimens taken from untreated gout patients by Watts et al. (1971), who also described crystals of hypoxanthine, xanthine and oxypurinol in patients being treated with allopurinol. Controlled observations were designed to exclude artefacts associated with rapid cooling, but the study has been to some extent controversial.

Tissue Variation and Temporal Relationships

It is evident that tophi are formed much more frequently in some tissues and organs than in others. The reason for this variation is not understood.

Supersaturation of tissue fluids with monosodium urate appears to be a necessary but not sufficient precondition for crystal deposition. Beyond this, local factors are clearly important. Urate deposition tends to occur in tissues rich in proteoglycans, particularly cartilage, and other possible influences include temperature, pH, trauma, tissue damage, pre-existing osteoarthritis, and local variation in urate concentration. For example, the immunity of the central nervous system from tophaceous deposition may be partly attributable to the low concentration of urate in the cerebrospinal fluid (Kelley et al. 1969).

The temporal relationship of hyperuricaemia, acute gout and tophus formation is also of interest. Before modern drug therapy was available, Hench (1936) found that the formation of clinical tophi took place between 3 and 42 (mean 11.6) years after the onset of gouty arthritis. The influence of the degree and duration of hyperuricaemia is well illustrated by a patient who developed the classic features of the Lesch-Nyhan syndrome shortly after birth; diagnosis was confirmed by the demonstration of a virtually complete absence of erythrocyte hypoxanthine-guanine phosphoribosyl transferase (HGPRT). Serum uric acid concentration was in the region of 720 μmol/l (12.0 mg/100 ml), and urinary uric acid level was 10.8 mmol (1800 mg)/24 h,

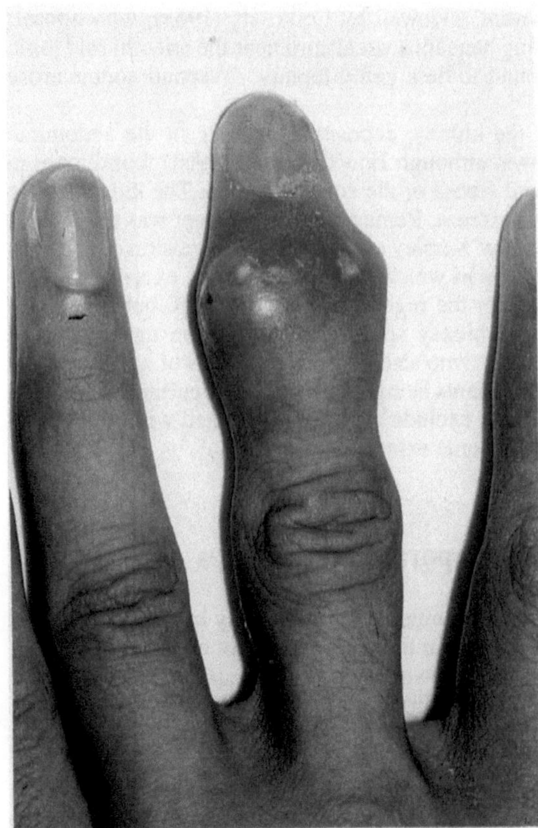

Fig. 9. Explosive onset of acute gout with tophaceous deposits in a young man with Lesch–Nyhan syndrome after 23 years of severe asymptomatic hyperuricaemia.

but for various reasons the parents decided that he should not receive allopurinol. For 23 years his gross hyperuricaemia remained untreated without the development of any joint symptoms – or, incidentally, any deterioration in renal function or evidence of urolithiasis. Then, suddenly, there was the explosive onset of polyarticular gout with deposition of numerous subcutaneous tophi (Fig. 9), events which the parents finally accepted as sufficient indications for treatment with allopurinol. Why had multifocal urate deposition and inflammation taken place so rapidly after such a long asymptomatic period?

The formation of chronic tophi before (or in the absence of) the development of acute gout was formerly regarded as a great rarity. It is sometimes seen in secondary gout associated with myeloproliferative diseases (Yü 1965) and in the Lesch-Nyhan syndrome (Wood et al. 1972) and was reported in a

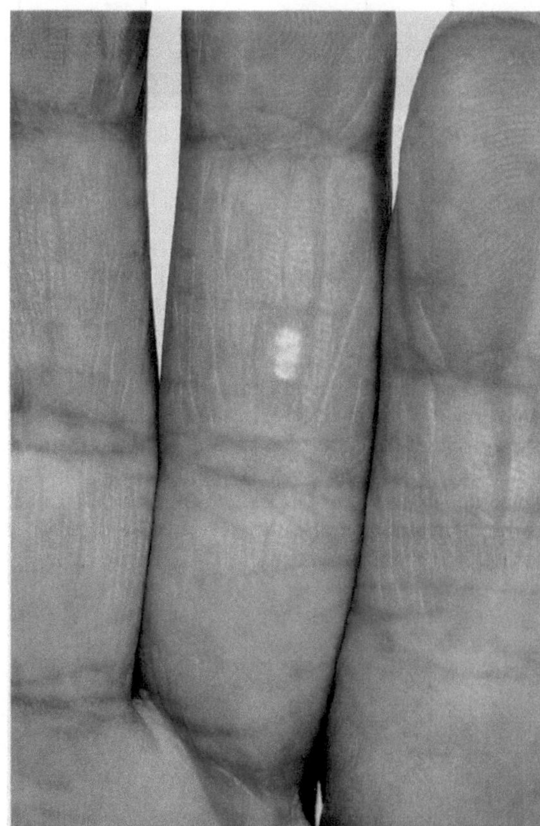

Fig. 10. Small cutaneous tophus in a patient who had never experienced acute gout. He had coincident rheumatoid arthritis and was receiving low doses of aspirin with resulting hyperuricaemia.

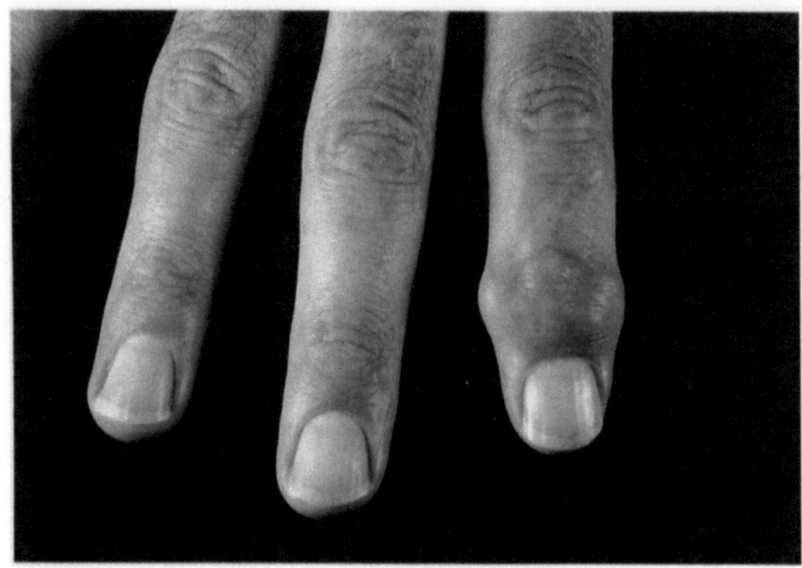

Fig. 11. Tophaceous deposit in a Heberden's node in a patient on long-term diuretic treatment.

bizarre case of primary juvenile gout (Smythe and Cutchin 1962). It is now perhaps seen more frequently. Hollingworth et al. (1983) described five such patients. One had co-existent rheumatoid arthritis (Fig. 10), and the other four showed various degrees of renal impairment; possible inhibitory factors in such situations upon acute gouty inflammation were discussed. However, all five patients were also taking urate-retaining drugs (diuretics or low-dose aspirin), and it is becoming apparent that the diuretic-induced gout often seen these days in elderly ladies sometimes takes the form of tophi in the absence of acute gout (Fig. 11) (Scott 1991). Such tophaceous deposits tend to be formed in association with Heberden's nodes at the distal interphalangeal joints, the white subcutaneous urate being visible in conjunction with bony osteophytes.

The Influence of Other Factors upon the Course of Chronic Gout

Apart from the actual deposition of urate within the tissues and organs described above, together with the kidney, brief consideration should be given to other associated factors, although a detailed discussion is not required in the present context.

It is generally accepted, and confirmed by Kahn (1976), that people with gout esteem their food highly, with eating and drinking being two of their greatest pleasures in life. Numerous epidemiological studies have shown a relationship betwen hyperuricaemia and body weight, and surveys of patients with gout have shown an increased prevalence of obesity – for example, 38% of subjects being more than 15% over their ideal body weights in the study of Grahame and Scott (1970). Loss of weight lowers the serum urate concentration (Emmerson 1973; Nichols and Scott 1972). Effects of alcohol upon hyperuricaemia and gout are complex: apart from the actual energy content of alcohol, it is likely that a high chronic intake produces increased synthesis of urate (Faller and Fox 1982) with acute intoxication providing an additional element of renal shutdown (MacLachlan and Rodnan 1967). Hypertriglyceridaemia is common in patients with gout: it may be that the association is due to the common factors of alcohol excess and obesity rather than to a direct causal mechanism (Gibson et al. 1979; Darlington 1984).

In accordance with other studies, Grahame and Scott (1970) found mild hypertension (defined as a diastolic blood pressure of between 91 and 130 mmHg) in 43% of their patients with gout and more severe hypertension in 9%. The incidence of hypertension was not related to disease duration, indicating that there is probably no added risk of developing hypertension with increasing duration of gout. The incidence of mild hypertension rose with advancing age of onset, but that of severe hypertension was highest in the decade 10–19 years, indicating the existence of a separate group of young subjects with gout, seveere hypertension and renal failure.

The problem of uric acid and vascular disease has attracted a large amount of work but remains to be clarified. In the Framingham survey (Hall et al. 1967), a relationship was found between the occurrence of gouty arthritis and signs of coronary artery disease, but on removal of patients with gout from the analysis any association between coronary disease and hyperuricaemia was no longer apparent. Neither male nor female with patients gout after presentation to hospital nor their male or female first-degree relatives were found to have an increased risk of dying from coronary artery or cardiovascular disease (Darlington et al. 1983). A trend towards an increased prevalence of coronary heart disease in hyperuricaemic subjects (Klein et al. 1973) was found to lack significance when the factors of body weight, hypertension and medication were taken into account.

Hyperuricaemia in the absence of such associations does not appear to be a coronary risk factor. Indeed, apart from special situations such as familial juvenile gout with renal disease (Calabrese et al. 1990) or HGPRT deficiency, the course of chronic gout is essentially benign when considered from the point of view of life-threatening disease, and life expectancy is not significantly reduced (Talbott and Lilienfeld 1959).

Urate Deposits in Asymptomatic Joints

In the early years of this century, Magnus-Levy (1909–1910) emphasised the fact that in many autopsies carried out on uraemic subjects, concretions were found in joints with no history of gout during life.

It has been generally accepted that an acute attack of gouty arthritis is provoked by the shedding or precipitation of crystals of monosodium urate into the synovial fluid (McCarty and Hollander 1961). Following resolution of the attack, however, crystals may still be found in the synovial fluid (Zwaifler and Pekin 1963) and membrane (Zevely et al. 1956; Schumacher and Kulka 1972). It has also been reported that metatarsophalangeal joints from previously uninvolved asymptomatic great toes could contain crystals of urate (Weinberger et al. 1979; Rouault et al. 1982), as could quiescent knee joints (Gordon et al. 1982).

The study of Kennedy et al. (1984) set out to investigate systematically the presence of crystals in the knee joints of 31 patients gout with who had never had an acute attack in that joint, concurrent examination of synovial fluid from the first toe (which had been the site of previous gout) also being performed. Crystalline material was seen on arthroscopy lying on the synovial membrane in 9 knees (28%) and confirmed histologically as monosodium urate in 4 (12.5%). Polarizing light microscopy of synovial fluid on 26 samples demonstrated urate crystals in 4 (12.5%) and calcium pyrophosphate dihydrate in 2 (6%). Fluid aspirated from 27 of the metatarsophalangeal joints revealed urate crystals in 14 (52%).

The mean serum uric acid concentration in patients in whom crystals were demonstrated was significantly higher than in the other patients. However, crystals were seen in four treated patients in whom very satisfactory control of the serum uric acid level had been achieved by treatment with allopurinol. In this context, a particularly instructive case (Scott 1978) was that of a man with severe polyarticular gout who became asymptomatic immediately his hyperuricaemia was corrected with allopurinol, but whose knee joint, examined by arthroscopy and biopsy before (Fig. 12) and again 6 months after (Fig. 13) the commencement of treatment, showed an apparently identical extent of urate deposition on both occasions.

Why then are attacks of gout transient and why do crystals not always produce inflammation? It is evident that urate-lowering treatment does not prevent attacks of gout merely by allowing crystals of urate to dissolve.

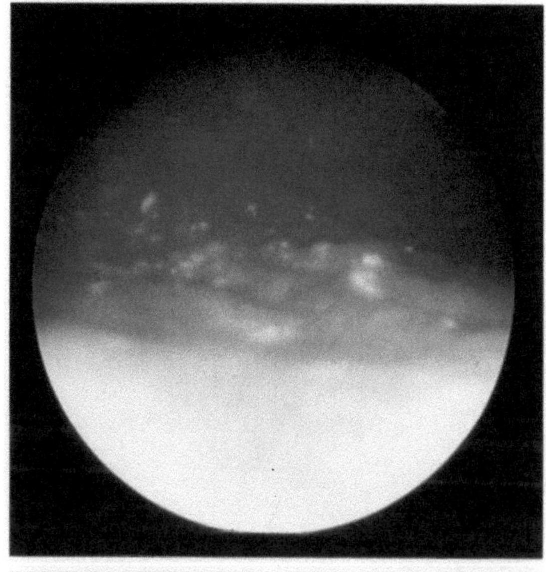

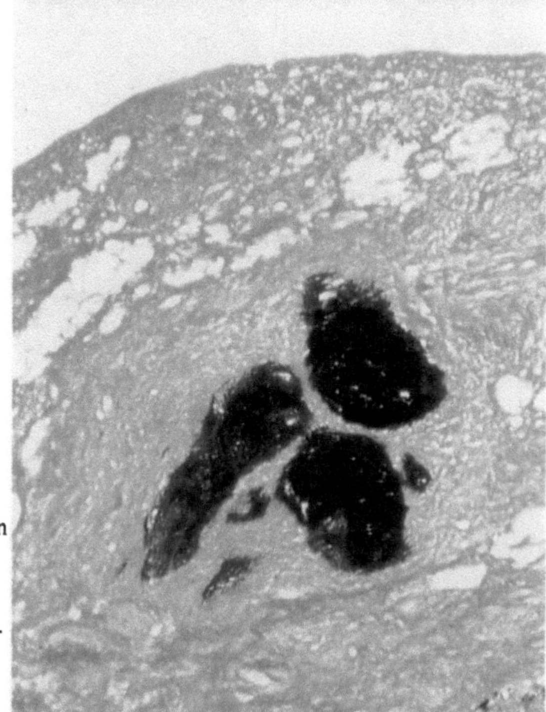

Fig. 12. (a) Arthroscopic appearance of knee joint in a patient with severe gout showing urate deposition on synovial membrane. (b) Synovial biopsy showing clumps of urate deposits (methenamine silver × 30).

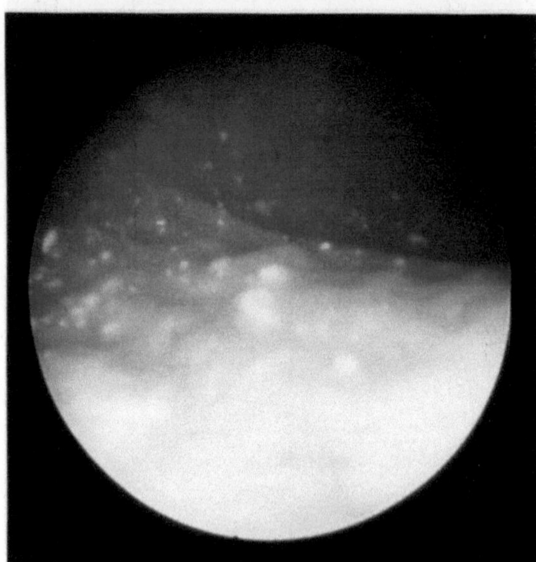

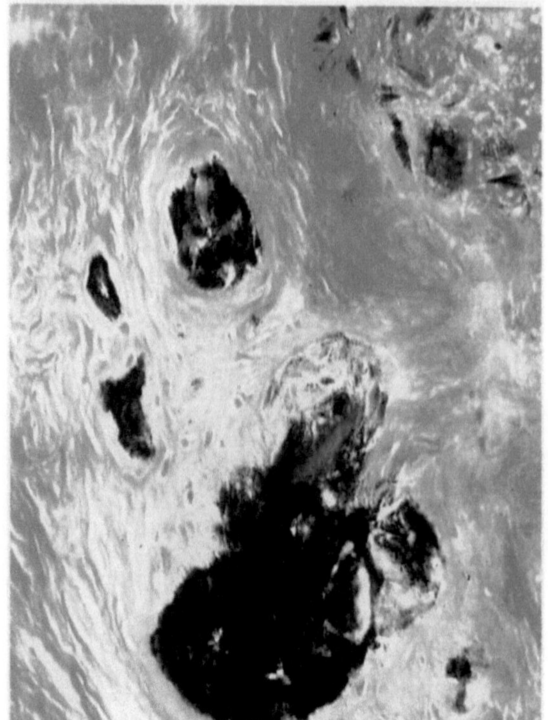

Fig. 13. Same patient as in Fig. 11, six months after he had become free of symptoms with Allopurinol treatment. (a) Arthroscopic appearance of knee joint, and (b) Synovial biopsy, showing little change from appearance before treatment.

Factors other than the mere presence of crystals are clearly necessary for the induction of inflammation. There has been speculation on influential properties of crystals such as shape, size, electrical charge and protein coating (Gordon et al. 1982; Tiliakos et al. 1980). Hernando et al. (1983), describing the transmission electron microscopic appearance of urate crystals, noted that despite diligent examination no protein-like coating was demonstrated on most crystals, but in their sole patient with asymptomatic gout a thick fluffy coating was observed. Of possible relevance to the case just cited is the finding of Malawista et al. (1979) that injury to cells exposed to silica crystals was related to the amount of dissolved urate in the experimental system.

Mechanisms of gouty inflammation are discussed elsewhere in this symposium. It should just be added that in the study of Kennedy et al. (1984) no particular aspect of crystal morphology (sharp or blunt, extracellular or intracellular) was observed. No clue was forthcoming as to why these little crystals – bland, dormant and innocuous – can at other times produce one of the most intense forms of pain known to man.

References

Bunim JJ, McEwen C (1940) Tophus of the mitral valve in gout. Arch Path 29: 700–704

Calabrese G, Simmonds HA, Cameron JS, Davies PM (1990) Precocious familial gout with reduced fractional urate clearance in normal purine enzymes. Quart J Med 75: 441–450

Champion D (1969) Gouty tenosynovitis and the carpal tunnel syndrome. Med J Australia 1: 1030–1032

Darlington LG (1984) Lean dry gout patients. Adv Exp Med Biol 165 A: 129–132

Darlington LG, Slack J, Scott JT (1983) Vascular mortality in patients with gout and their families. Ann Rheum Dis 42: 270–273

De Séze S, Ryckewaert A, Levernieux J, Marteau R (1958) Physiopathology, clinical manifestations and treatment of gout. Part 2. Clinical and therapeutic studies. Ann Rheum Dis 17: 15–21

De Sèze S, Phankim-Koupernik M (1964) Syndrome du canal carpien d'origine goutteuse. Revue de Rhumatisme et des Maladies Osteo-Articulaires 31: 9–12

Edwards WG, Lincoln CR, Basset FH et al. (1969) The tarsal tunnel syndrome. JAMA 207: 716–720

Emmerson BT (1966) Alteration in urate metabolism by weight reduction. Aus & NZ J Med 3: 410–437

Faller J, Fox IH (1982) Ethanol-induced hyperuricemia. Evidence for increased urate production by activation of adenine nucleotide turnover. N Eng J Med 307: 1598–1602

Fishman RS, Sunderman FW (1966) Band keratopathy in gout. Arch Ophthal 75: 367–369

Frauenfelder FT, Hanna C, Dreis MW, Cosgrove KW (1982) Cataracts associated with allopurinol therapy. Am J Ophthalmol 94: 137–209

Gawoski JM, Balogh K, Landis WJ (1985) Aortic-valvular tophus: identification by X-ray diffraction of urate and calcium phosphates. J Clin Path 38: 873–876

Gibson T, Kilbourn K, Horner I, Simmonds HA (1979) Mechanism and treatment of hypertriglyceridaemia in gout. Ann Rheum Dis 38: 31–35

Gordon TP, Bertouch JV, Walsh BR, Brooks PM (1982) Monosodium urate crystals in asymptomatic knee joints. J Rheumatol 9: 967–969

Grahame R, Scott JT (1970) Clinical survey of 354 patients with gout. Ann Rheum Dis 29: 461–468

Gutman AB (1973) The past four decades of progress in the knowledge of gout, with an assessment of the present status. Arth Rheum 16: 431–445

Hall AP, Barry PE, Dawber T, McNamara PM (1967) Epidemiology of gout and hyperuricemia. Amer J Med 42: 27–37

Hall MC, Selin G (1960) Spinal involvement in gout. J Bone Joint Surg 42 A: 341–343

Hawkins CF, Ellis HA, Rawson A (1965) Malignant gout with tophaceous small intestine and megaloblastic anaemia. Ann Rheum Dis 24: 224–233

Hench PS (1936) The diagnosis of gout and gouty arthritis. J Lab Clin Med 220: 48–55

Hench PS, Darnall CM (1933) A clinic on acute, old-fashioned gout; with special reference to its inciting factors. Med Clin N Amer 16: 1371–1393

Hernando P, Reginato AJ, Schumacher HR (1983) Morphological characteristics of sodium urate: a transmission electron microscopic study of intact natural and synthetic crystals. Ann Rheum Dis 42: 75–81

Hollingworth P, Scott JT, Burry HC (1983) Non-articular gout: hyerpuricaemia and thophus formation without gouty arthritis. Arth Rheum 26: 98–101

Hunder GG, Worthington JW, Bickel WM (1968) Avascular necrosis of the femoral head in a patient with gout. JAMA 203: 47–49

Kahn MF (1976) Goutte, obésite et plaisirs de la table. Comparison entre 40 goutteux et 40 témoins. Nouvelle Presse Medicale 5: 1897–1898

Kelley WN, Greene ML, Rosenbloom JF et al. (1969) Hypoxanthine-guaninine phosphoribosyltransferase deficiency in gout. Ann Int Med 70: 155–206

Kennedy TD, Higgens CS, Woodrow DF, Scott JT (1984) Crystal deposition in the knee and great toe joints of asymptomatic gout patients. J Roy Soc Med 77: 747–750

Kersley GD, Mandel L, Jeffrey MR (1950) Gout. An unusual case with softening and subluxation of the first cervical vertebra and splenomegaly. Ann Rheum Dis 9: 282–304

Klein R, Klein BE, Cornono et al. (1973) Serum uric acid. Its relation to coronary heart disease risk factors and cardiovascular disease. Arch Int Med 132: 401–410

Koskoff YD, Morris LE, Lubic LG (1953) Paraplegia as a complication of gout. JAMA 152: 37–38

Lagier R, MacGee W (1983) Spondylodiscal erosions due to gout: anatomicoradiological study of a case. Ann Rheum Dis 42: 350–353

Lefkovits AM (1965) Gouty involvement of the larynx. Report of a case and review of the literature. Arth Rheum 8: 1019–1026

Lichtenstein L, Scott HW, Levin MH (1956) Pathologic changes in gout. Survey of 11 necropsied cases. Amer J Path 32: 871–895

Litvak J, Briney W (1973) Extradural spinal depositions of urates producing paraplegia. J Neurosurg 39: 656–658

Liu CSC, Brown NAP, Leonard TJK, Bull PW, Scott JT (1988) Cataract in allopurinol treatment. Eye 2: 600–606

McCarty DJ, Hollander JL (1961) Identification of urate crystals in gouty synovial fluid. Ann Int Med 54: 452–460

McCollum DE, Mathews RS, O'Neil MT (1970) Aseptic necrosis of the femoral head: associated diseases and evaluation of treatment. Southern Med J 63: 241–253

MacLachlan MJ, Rodnan GP (1967) Effects of food, fast and alcohol on serum uric acid and acute attacks of gout. Amer J Med 42: 38–57

McWilliams JR (1952) Ocular findings in gout. Amer J Ophthalmol 35: 1778–1783

Magid SK, Gray CE, Anand A (1981) Spinal canal compression by tophi in a patient with chronic polyarthritis: case report and literature review. Arth Rheum 24: 1431–1434

Magnus-Levy A (1909–1910) quoted by Sokoloff L (1957)

Mahapatro RC, Sylvia LC, Becker SM (1985) Intraosseous gouty tophus. J Med Soc New Jersey 82: 41–42

Malawista SE, Van Blaricom G, Cretella SB, Schwartz ML (1979) The phlogistic potential of urate in solution. Studies of the phagocytic process in human leukocytes. Arth Rheum 22: 728–736

Malawista SE, Seegmiller JR, Hathaway BC, Sokoloff L (1965) Sacroiliac gout. JAMA 194: 954–956

Nicholls A, Scott JT (1972) Effect of weight loss on plasma and urinary levels of uric acid. Lancet 2: 1223–1224

Perricone E, Brandt KD (1978) Enhancement of urate solubility by connective tissue. Arth Rheum 21: 453–460

Pund EE, Hawley RL, McGee HJ, Blount SG (1960) Gouty Heart. N Eng J Med 263: 835–838

Rotes Querol AJ, Munoz Gomez GJ (1965) Gota en la ladera. Rev Espan do reumatismo y enfermedades osteoarticulares 11: 89–98

Rouault T, Caldwell DA, Holmes EW (1982) Aspiration of the asymptomatic metatarsophalangeal joint in gout patients and hyperuricemic controls. Arth Rheum 25: 209–212

Scalapino JN, Edwards WD, Steckelberg JM et al. (1984) Mitral stenosis associated with valvular tophi. Mayo Clin Proc 59: 509–512

Schumacher HR, Kulka JP (1972) Needle biopsy of synovial membrane – experience with the Parker-Pearson technic. New Eng J Med 286: 416–419

Scott JT (1978) New knowledge of the pathogenesis of gout. J Clin Path 12 (Suppl): 205–213

Scott JT (1991) Drug-induced gout. Baillière's Clinical Rheumatology, Vol. 5, No 1: 39–60

Sequeira W, Bouffard AB, Salgia K, Skosey J (1981) Quadriparesis in tophaceous gout. Arth Rheum 24: 1442–1444

Serre H, Simone L, Claustre J (1963) A propos de l'atteinte des hanches au cours de goutte. Revue du rhumatisme 19: 363–390

Smythe CM, Cutchin JH (1962) Primary juvenile gout. Amer J Med 32: 799–804

Slansky HH, Kuwabara T (1968) Intranuclear urate crystals in corneal epithelium. Arch Ophthalmol 80: 338–344

Sokoloff L (1957) The pathology of gout. Metabolism 6: 230–243

Stockman A, Darlington LG, Scott JT (1980) Frequency of chondrocalcinosis of the knees and avascular necrosis of the femoral heads in gout: a controlled study. Ann Rheum Dis 39: 7–11

Tiliakos N, Goldman JA, Wilson CH, Rajapakse D (1980) Intrasynovial sodium changes in gout. Arth Rheum 23: 756 (abstract)
Talbott JH, Lilienfeld A (1959) Longevity in gout. Geriatrics 14: 409–420
Traut EF, Knight AA, Szanto PB, Passerelli EW (1954) Specific vascular changes in gout. JAMA 156: 591–593
Varga J, Giampaolo C, Goldenberg DL (1985) Tophaceous gout of the spine in a patient with no peripheral tophi: case report and review of the literature. Arth Rheum 28: 1312–1315
Vinstein AL, Cockerill EM (1972) Involvement of the spine in gout. Radiology 103: 311–312
Virtanen KSI, Halonen PI (1969) Total heart block as a complication of gout. Cardiologia 54: 359–363
Wald SL, McLennan JE, Carroll RM, Segal H (1979) Extradural spinal involvement by gout. J Neurosurg 50: 236–239
Watts RWE, Scott JT, Chalmers RA et al. (1971) Microscopic studies on skeletal muscle in gout patients treated with allopurinol. Quart J Med 40: 1–14
Weinberger A, Schumacher HR, Agudelo C (1979) Urate crystals in asymptomatic metatarsophalangeal joints. Ann Int Med 91: 56–57
Wood MD, Fox RM, Vincent L, Rege C, O'Sullivan WJ (1972) The Lesch-Nyhan syndrome: report of three cases. Aust NZ J Med 1: 57–64
Yü T-F (1965) Secondary gout associated with myeloproliferative disease. Arth Rheum 8: 765–771
Yü T-F (1974) Milestones in the treatment of gout. Amer J Med 56: 676–685
Zevely HA, French AJ, Mikklesen WM, Duft IF (1956) Synovial specimens obtained by knee joint punch biopsy. Amer J Med 20: 510–519
Zvaifler NJ, Pekin TJ (1963) Significance of urate crystals in synovial fluids. Arch Int Med 111: 99–102

Questions and Comments Raised for Discussion

J. G. Puig

An increased urate pool, if untreated, is thought to progress from asymptomatic hyperuricemia, through intermittent episodes of acute gouty arthritis, to chronic tophaceous gout (CTG). In recent years, however, two facts have cast some doubt on the consistency of this statement. First, several clinical descriptions and studies have documented that CTG does not always produce articular crippling deformities. In fact, tophaceous changes usually appear in bones before MSU deposits are observed on physical examination [1]. Thus, in some cases only a complete radiographic examination will reveal articular or bone lesions due to gout (i. e. sacroiliac lesions). Second, CTG may not be preceded by symptomatic recurrent articular inflammatory episodes [2]. MSU crystals do not always elicit an inflammatory response demanding medical attention, although in most cases these deposits do cause a subclinical response that may finally end in bone and/or articular damage. In fact, patients with CTG have been reported in whom no episodes of acute arthritis could be documented. Postmenopausal hypertensive women with decreased renal function are a paradigmatic example of "unusual CTG"; either because they present unusual tophi locations or because asymptomatic CTG is casually diagnosed. In some cases this form of CTG is neither expressed by articular deformities nor is it the result of recurrent inflammatory arthritis ("unusual CTG"). The true incidence, location and pathophysiologic response of asymptomatic MSU deposits is poorly known. We need to define better the clinical characteristics of "unusual CTG." For instance, the association between nodal osteoarthritis and MSU deposition has been recognized only recently. A number of in vitro experiments, such as the finding that a high Ca^{2+} concentration increases MSU nucleation, have prompted several hypotheses to explain this association. An affirmative answer to the question of whether the increased bone reabsorption of postmenopausal women facilitates MSU deposits would partially explain the predominance of postmenopausal women among the female gouty population and the increased prevalence and different location of tophi in gouty women when compared to men with gout [3].

In contrast to other crystal-deposition diseases, the extraordinary benefits that could be obtained from hypouricemic therapy should stimulate the early detection of tophi which could influence therapeutic recommendations.

References

1. Nakayama DA, Barthelemy C, Carrera G, Lightfoot RW, Wortman RL (1984) Tophaceous gout: a clinical and radiographic assessment. Arthritis Rheum 27: 468–471
2. Shmerling RH, Stern SH, Gravellese EM, Kantrowitz FG (1988) Thopaceous deposition in the finger pads without gouty arthritis. Arch Intern Med 148: 1830–1832
3. Puig JG, Michán AD, Jiménez ML et al. (1990) Female gout: clinical spectrum and uric acid metabolism. Arch Intern Med (in press)

LÖFFLER

I have an example of a positive technetium scan of a soft-tissue tophus here. However, a tophus might well behave like, for example, a bone lesion due to plasmocytoma: Whenever there is an inflammatory reaction due to increase in size of the lesion, the scan will be positive, whereas during a period of stability with inflammatory response having subsided, the scan may be negative for tophi in bone as well as soft tissue.

K. L. SCHMIDT

Is it possible to detect tophi, especially in the bone, by scintigraphy? How do the scans look? Are there differences between more inflamed and more "destructive" (osteolytic) tophi?

9

The Course of Chondrocalcinosis

M. SCHATTENKIRCHNER

The term "chondrocalcinosis" means a descriptive diagnosis of calcium deposition in joint cartilage, which is not further specified. From this etymological view, chondrocalcinosis therefore is a pathomorphological or at most a roentgenological diagnosis. However, the term chondrocalcinosis was coined by clinicians. In 1958, Zitnan and Sitaj described the clinical and roentgenological features of what they called in Latin *chondrocalcinosis articularis*. They described the features of cases of a hereditary arthropathy with calcium deposits in the joint cartilage.

In 1962, McCarty and co-workers identified calcium phosphate crystals both in the synovial fluid and in the cartilage of arthritic patients with the so-called pseudogout syndrome. Since then, chondrocalcinosis has been used both as a roentgenological and a clinical diagnosis, the latter as a synonym of calcium pyrophosphate dihydrate (CPPD) arthropathy.

In their earliest observations in 1962 of patients with CPPD arthropathy, McCarty and co-workers concluded that there must be various clinical manifestations of this disturbance. They described acute gout-like attacks as well as various forms of chronic arthritis.

Frequency and Classification of Chondrocalcinosis

Little is known about the frequency of chondrocalcinosis. There is a strong correlation between increasing frequency of chondrocalcinosis and ageing, both in roentgenological and in pathomorphological studies. Mohr (1984) has summarised data concerning this topic from all available studies in two tables (Tables 1, 2). According to the presence or absence of recognised predisposing factors, chondrocalcinosis can be classified as hereditary, associated with metabolic disease or sporadic (vel idiopathic) (Table 3). The sporadic form is by far the most common one encountered.

Hereditary cases mostly show a polyarticular form of early arthritis in the 3rd to 5th decade of life. Also, patients with chondrocalcinosis associated with metabolic disorders tend to present with roentgenological or clinical manifestations at an earlier age than the idiopathic form. In some metabolic forms which also have an increasing frequency with advancing age, it is difficult to judge whether there is a biochemical relation to chondrocalcinosis

Table 1. Frequency of roentgenologically apparent chondrocalcinosis

Localisation	Age (years)	Frequency	Reference
Disc	–	Very rare	Lusskin 1927
Disc	Adult	Very frequent	De Sèze et al. 1956
Meniscus	–	0.3%	Wolke 1935
Meniscus	$\bar{x} = 80$	7%	Bocher et al. 1965
Meniscus	60–94 90–94	6.1% 13.6%	Cabanel et al. 1970
Meniscus	80–99 ($\bar{x} = 88.4$ ♀)	23.1%	Memin et al. 1978
Wrist	41–91 (♂) ($\bar{x} = 79.7$ ♂)	2% 5%	Trentham et al. 1975
Knee	$\bar{x} = 78$ >85	34% 47%	Wilkins et al. 1981
Knee	$\bar{x} = 68.25$	6.9%	Moalla et al. 1981
Various joints	$\bar{x} = 84.3$ >70	27.6% 32%	Ellman and Levin 1975
Various joints	<79 >80	13% 37.7%	Emériau et al. 1977
Various joints	$\bar{x} = 85$ >90	32% 60%	Delauche et al. 1977
Various joints	$\bar{x} = 78$ 65–74 75–84 >85	34% 11% 35% 47%	Wilkins et al. 1981

(Mohr 1984)

Table 2. Frequency of morphologically proven calcium pyrophosphate dihydrate deposition

Localisation	Age (years)	Frequency	Reference
Disc	55–59	10%	Mohr et al. 1979
Disc	15–80	3.1%	Lagier and Wildi 1979
Meniscus	11–74	2%	Aufdermaur and Lentzsch 1979
Meniscus	$\bar{x} = 73.5$ (♂) $\bar{x} = 81.5$ (♀)	18.6% 30.6%	Mitrovic et al. 1981

(Mohr 1984)

Table 3. Classification of calcium pyrophosphate dihydrate crystal deposition disease

I. Hereditary
   A. Czechoslovakian
   B. Chilean
   C. Dutch
   D. Other

II. Sporadic (idiopathic)

III. Associated with metabolic disease
   A. Hyperparathyroidism
   B. Haemochromatosis
   C. Hypothyroidism
   D. Gout
   E. Other (ochronosis, Wilson's disease, diabetes mellitus, hypophosphatasia)
   F. Ageing

(McCarty 1976)

Table 4. Metabolic conditions that predispose to calcium pyrophosphate dihydrate crystal deposition

Definite associations

Hyperparathyroidism (Pritchard and Jessop 1977)
Haemochromatosis (Hamilton et al. 1981)
Gout (Hollingworth et al. 1982)
Hypophosphatasia (Eade et al. 1981)
Hypomagnesaemia (Runeberg et al. 1975)

Probable associations

Hypothyroidism (Alexander et al. 1982)
Ochronosis (Schumacher and Holdsworth 1977)
Wilson's disease (Feller and Schumacher 1972)
Senile amyloid (Ryan et al. 1982)

(Doherty and Dieppe 1986)

or only a concurrence of two common age-related conditions. For diabetes, uraemia and Paget's disease the latter was shown by McCarty et al. (1974) and Boussina et al. (1976).

Doherty and Dieppe have listed all information from studies concerning metabolic conditions that predispose to CPPD crystal deposition. They divide these conditions into definite and probable associations (Table 4).

In clinical practice it has proved a good rule that every case of roentgenologically apparent chondrocalcinosis or of pseudogout syndrome in a patient under 50 years of age should be suspected as being associated with a metabolic disease or with a hereditary form of chondrocalcinosis.

Table 5. Classification of clinical manifestations according to McCarty (1975)

		Frequency
Type A	Pseudogout (isolated)	8.9%[a]
B	Pseudorheumatoid arthritis	5.4%
C and D	Pseudo-osteoarthritis (with and without inflammatory attacks of pseudogout)	66.9%
E	Lanthanic (asymptomatic) calcium pyrophosphate deposits	5.4%
F	Pseudoneurotrophic	13.5%

[a] Numbers are taken (according to Mohr 1984) from Menkes et al. (1976)

Table 6. Classification of clinical manifestations according to Fallet (1989)

	Frequency
1. Acute mono- or oligoarthritis (pseudogout)	25%
2. Relapsing inflammatory polyarthropathy	5%
3. Chronic arthralgia (exclusively women)	50%
4. Destructive mono-, oligo- or polyarticular arthropathy ($♀ > ♂$)	20%

Table 7. Classification of clinical manifestations according to Doherty and Dieppe (1986)

1. Pseudogout (acute CPPD-induced synovitis)
2. Chronic CPPD arthropathy

CPPD, calcium pyrophosphate dihydrate

Clinical Patterns of Arthritis and Course of Chondrocalcinosis

Only a few clinical surveys of patients with nonhereditary chondrocalcinosis exist; epidemiologic data are lacking. In most series women predominate. The mean age at clinical manifestation is about 65–75 years.

According to clinical manifestations and course, three classifications were elaborated and proposed for clinical use by McCarty et al. (1975; Table 5), Fallet (1989; Table 6) and Doherty and Dieppe (1986; Table 7).

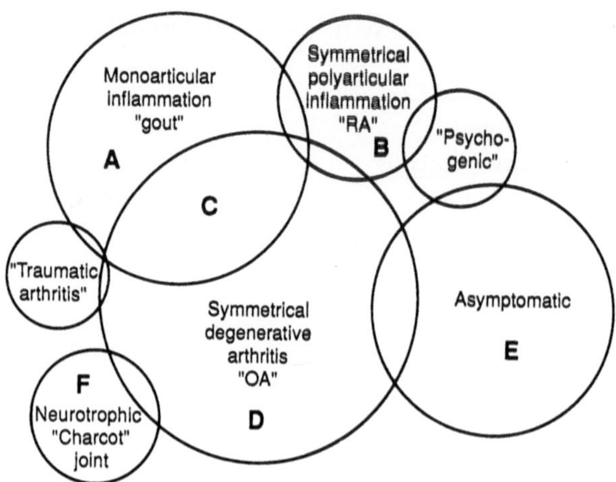

Fig. 1. Arthritis patterns of joint involvement in CPPD arthropathies (McCarty 1974)

To elucidate the diagnostic mimicry in arthritis patterns, McCarty published a diagrammatic presentation of diagnosis commonly given to patients with articular CPPD crystal deposits (Fig. 1).

Open Questions Concerning the Development and Course of Chondrocalcinosis

Neither a common biochemical way in the different kinds of chondrocalcinosis nor a single way in a special form of chondrocalcinosis which leads to the roentgenological or clinical manifestations of this disorder is well-defined.

Both local matrix changes (biochemical- or morphological-like matrix vesicles described by Anderson 1988) and systemic conditions (as postulated by Katz 1975 in gouty inflammation) could be responsible for initiating the disease process.

Interesting results were published by Hamilton et al. in measuring the inorganic pyrophosphate content in synovial fluid. They found a significant elevation of the inorganic pyrophosphate level in haemochromatosis, hypomagnesaemia and hyperparathyroidism. In patients with hypothyroidism – a disease with a questionable role as a predisposing factor for CPPD arthropathy – lower values than in normal subjects were measured.

Nothing is known about the course of lanthanic or asymptomatic chondrocalcinosis. Neither do we know the factors which lead to an acute pseudo-

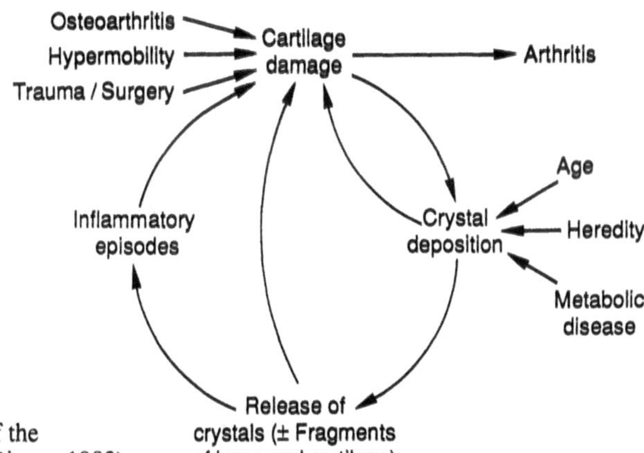

Fig. 2. Hypothesis of the amplification loop (Dieppe 1982)

gout attack or to one of the different forms of chronic or chronically relapsing oligo- or polyarthritis.

We do not understand the conditions for the development of polyarticular or mono- or oligoarticular involvement or of the involvement of small or big joints.

In a group of 35 patients with idiopathic haemochromatosis 22 suffered from an arthropathy, in 20 in the metacarpophalangeal joints. Four had chondrocalcinosis of a big joint (knee or wrist), two in combination with metacarpophalangeal arthropathy, two isolated (Schattenkirchner et al. 1983). Not any criteria could be found including HLA pattern which correlated to joint manifestations or joint pattern of manifestation in this group with idiopathic haemochromatosis. One observation also made by others was the non-response on iron-depletion therapy. On the contrary, one patient experienced a first joint attack after the beginning of treatment.

The reasons are unclear why there is joint destruction in one group of arthropathies and hypertrophic bone changes in others. The co-existence of CPPD and hydroxyapatite crystals in synovial fluids of patients with osteoarthritis has been associated with clinically more severe joint destruction when compared with synovial fluids containing crystals of only one type. In animal experiments, however, Watanabe et al. (1990) could not affirm this observation.

The high frequency of mechanical joint lesions in patients with chondrocalcinosis motivated Dieppe to his hypothesis of an "amplification loop", which states that joint damage is one of several mechanisms that predispose to CPPD crystal formation (Fig. 2). CPPD arthropathy is usually associated with a hypertrophic bone response. Thus, the many different forms and

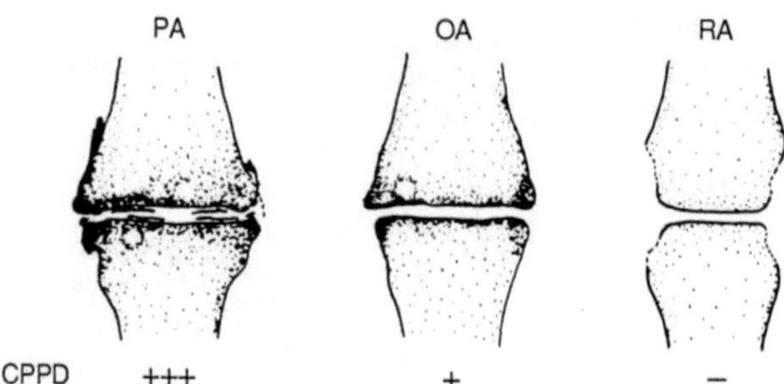

Fig. 3. CPPD crystal deposition and bone response (Doherty and Dieppe 1986). *PA*, primary arthritis; *OA*, osteoarthritis; and *RA*, rheumatoid arthritis

courses of arthropathy in which CPPD crystals can be detected or chondrocalcinosis can be seen roentgenologically could be explained according to Doherty and Dieppe (1986) as a superimposition of CPPD disease processes on other disease patterns, supposedly most frequently on systemic (primary) or secondary osteoarthritis, perhaps also on other crystal-induced arthropathies such as gout or hydroxyapatite disease (Fig. 3).

In summary, many clinical phenomena in chondrocalcinosis are unexplained. I could emphasize the large variety of clinical manifestations of CPPD arthropathy rather than describe the natural course of the different forms.

References

Alexander GM, Dieppe PA, Doherty M, Scott DG (1982) Pyrophosphate arthropathy: a study of metabolic associations and laboratory parameters. Ann Rheum Dis 41: 377–381

Anderson HC (1988) Mechanisms of pathologic calcification. In: McCarty DJ (ed) Crystalline deposition diseases. Rheum Dis Clin North America, Vol 14. WB Saunders, Philadelphia, London, Toronto, Montreal, Sydney, Tokyo, p 303–319

Aufdermaur M, Lentzsch S (1979) Die Chondrocalcinose (Pseudogicht) des Kniegelenkmeniskus. Dtsch Med Wschr 104: 1166–1171

Bocher J, Mankin HJ, Berk RN, Rodnan GP (1965) Prevalence of calcified meniscal cartilage in elderly persons. New Engl J Med 272: 1093–1097

Boussina I, Gerster JC, Epiney J, Fallet GH (1976) A study of the incidence of articular chondrocalcinosis in Paget's disease of bone. Scand J Rheumatol 5: 33–35

Cabanel G, Phelip X, Verdier JM, Gras J-P (1970) Fréquence des calcifications méniscales et leur signification pathologique. Rhumatologie 7: 255–262

Delauche MC, Stehle B, Cassou B, Verret JM, Kahn ML (1977) Fréquence de la chondrocalcinose radiologique après 80 ans. Rev Rhum 44: 556–557

De Séze S, Dijan A, Claisse R (1956) La discopathie calcificante. Rev Rhum 25: 265–281

Dieppe PA, Alexander GM, Jones H (1982) Pyrophosphate arthropathy: a clinical and radiological study of 105 cases. Ann Rheum Dis 41: 371–376

Doherty M, Dieppe P (1986) Crystal deposition disease in the elderly. In: Clinics in rheumatic diseases. Kean WF (ed) Arthritis in the elderly. Vol 12, pp 97–116

Eade AWT, Swannell AJ, Williamson N (1981) Pyrosphosphate arthropathy in hypophosphatasia. Ann Rheum Dis 40: 164–170

Ellman MH, Levin B (1975) Chondrocalcinosis in elderly persons. Arthritis Rheum 18: 43–47

Emériau JP, Borde C, Chapoulart H, Bruneton J-N, De Sèze M, Galley P, Tavernier J, Choussat H (1977) Chondrocalcinose articulaire asymptomatique chez le sujet agé. Bordeaux méd 10: 825–830

Fallet GH (1989) Chondrokalzinose. In: Fehr K, Miehle W, Schattenkirchner M, Tillmann K: Rheumatologie in Praxis und Klinik. Thieme, Stuttgart, New York, pp 9.19–9.29

Feller ER, Schumacher HR (1972) Osteoarticular changes in Wilson's disease. Arthritis Rheum 15: 259–266

Hamilton EBD, Bomford AB, Laws JW, Williams R (1981) The natural history of arthritis in idiopathic haemochromatosis: progression of the clinical and radiological features over ten years. Quart J Med 199: 321–329

Hollingworth P, Williams PL, Scott JT (1982) Frequency of chondrocalcinosis of the knees in asymptomatic hyperuricaemia and rheumatoid arthritis: a controlled study. Ann Rheum Dis 41: 344–346

Katz WA (1975) Deposition of urate crystals in gout. Altered connective tissue metabolism. Arthritis Rheum 18 (Suppl): 751–756

Lagier R, Wildi E (1979) Fréquence de la chondrocalcinose dans une serie de 1000 disques intervertebraux excisés chirurgicalement. Rev Rhum 46 (1979) 303–307

Lusskin H (1927) Calcified intervertebral disk. Amer J Surg 3: 148–149

McCarty DJ, Kohn NN, Faires JS (1962) The significance of calcium phosphate crystals in the synovial fluid of arthritis patients: the "pseudogout syndrome" I. Clinical aspects. Ann Intern Med 56: 711–737

McCarty DJ (1974) Diagnostic mimicry in arthritis – patterns of joint involvement associated with calcium pyrophosphate dihydrate crystal deposits. Bull Rheum Dis 25: 804–809

McCarty DJ, Silcox DC, Coe F (1974) Diseases associated with calcium pyrophosphate dihydrate crystal deposition. A controlled study. Amer J Med 56: 704–714

McCarty DJ (1976) Calcium pyrophosphate dihydrate crystal deposition disease – 1975. Arthritis Rheum 19: 275–285

Memin Y, Monville C, Ryckewaert (1978) La chondrocalcinosis articulaire après 80 ans. Rev Rhum 45: 77–82

Menkes CJ, Simon F, Delrien F, Forest M, Debarre F (1976) Destructive arthropathy in chondrocalcinosis articularis. Arthritis Rheum 19: 329–348

Mitrovic D, Stankovic A, Morin J, Bard M, Memin Y, de Sèze S, Ryckewaert A (1981) Meniscal and cartilagenous calcifications in the knee joint of 127 cadavers. Rev Rhum N spéc, Abstr. Nr 831

Moalla M, Hamza M, Ben Ayed H (1981) Epidemiologie de la chondrocalcinose en Tunisie. Rev Rhum, Numéro spécial, Abs. Nr. 834

Mohr W (1984) Arthritiden durch körpereigene Stoffwechselprodukte (mikrokristalline Arthritiden). In: Mohr W (ed) Gelenkkrankheiten. Thieme, Stuttgart, New York, pp 40–67

Mohr W, Oehler K, Hersener J, Wilke W (1979) Chondrocalcinose der Zwischenwirbelscheiben. Z Rheumatol 38: 11–26

Pritchard MH, Jessop JD (1977) Chondrocalcinosis in primary hyperthyroidism. Influence of age, metabolic bone disease and parathyroidectomy. Ann Rheum Dis 36: 146–151

Runeberg L, Collan Y, Jokinen EJ, Lahdevirta J, Aro A (1975) Hypomagnesaemia due to renal disease of unknown etiology. Amer J Med 59: 873–881

Ryan LM, Liang G, Kozin F (1982) Amyloid arthropathy: possible association with chondrocalcinosis. J Rheum 9: 273–278

Schattenkirchner M, Fischbacher L, Giebner-Fischbacher U, Albert ED (1983) Arthropathie bei der idiopathischen Hämochromatose. Klin Wochenschr 61: 1199–1207

Schumacher HR, Holdsworth DE (1977) Ochronotic arthropathy I. Clinicopathologic studies. Sem Arthr Rheum 6: 207–246

Trentham DE, Masi AT, Hamm RL (1975) Roentgenographic prevalence of chondrocalcinosis. Arthritis Rheum 18: 627–628

Watanabe W, Baker DG, Schumacher HR Jr (1990) Comparison of the acute inflammation induced by calcium pyrophosphate dihydrate (CPPD), apatite (AP) and mixed crystals in the rat air pouch model of a synovial space. Arthritis Rheum 33 (Suppl): S54 (Abstr.)

Wilkins E, Dieppe PA, Maddison P, Eveson G (1981) Chondrocalcinosis and osteoarthritis in the elderly. Rev Rhum Numéro special, Abstr Nr. 832

Wilkins E, Dieppe PA, Maddison P, Eveson G (1981) Articular chondrocalcinosis and its association with osteoarthritis in the elderly. Ann Rheum Dis 40: 516 (Abstr.)

Wolke K (1935) Über Meniskus- und Gelenkknorpelverkalkungen. Acta radiol 16: 577–588

Zitnan D, Sitaj S (1958) Mnohopocetna familiarha Kalcifikaciz artikularynch chrupiek. Bratisl Lek Listy 38: 217–228

Questions and Comments Raised for Discussion

LÖFFLER

There is one disease which deserves special consideration with respect to pathophysiology of CaPPD crystal deposition. In the inborn error of bone metabolism, hypophosphatasia, pyrophosphate concentrations in body fluids are well in excess of what has been measured in any other disease. However, children with this defect will rarely or never develop CaPPD deposition, while about 40%–50% of adult patients do. Comparing findings in adult patients with and without CaPPD deposition might give us some clue as to which factors other than pyrophosphate are or are not important contributors to CaPPD deposition.

10

Round Table Discussion

WATTS:
And I would like to start this session on treatment by drawing your attention
to one of the few things which I think have not been discussed here. This is
namely the possible role of hyperuricemia in oxalate stone disease. You will
of course all be aware of the ability of calculi to form in the calcium oxalate
model and dyhydrate crystals to grow on either uric acid or uric acid dyhydrate crystals by virtuexpitexy and because of uricacid as one of the risk
factors which Robertson and his colleagues recognized for oxalate stone
disease and this has of course given rise to the test of where one has very
recurrent oxylate stone disease, inhipathic oxylate stone disease, one could
perhaps profitably contempt to reduce the urine uricacid level. And, I must
say this is my opinion, my own opinion, which I will throw out for purpose of
this discussion and perhaps to raise a litte controversy, that Allopurinol has
certainly not become the routine treatment or patients with idiopathic stone
disease although it can be justified in a few patients who got in fact a urisasis
which is not being relieved by hydration, a lower oxylate, low vitamin, low
calcium, low-purin diet. So, has anybody any views upon this question of
recurrent idiopathic calcium oxylate stone disease in relation to the possibly
controlling the nucleation by keepin the uricacid very low. I think the situation is different where you demonstrate the high urine uricacid, where you
begin with the normal level of uricacid. Is this a logical thing to do or not?
I think this is Dr. Puig raises a little bit, yesterday.

PUIG:
Thank you, Dr. Watts. First of all, at our stone clinic we have worked for
some years on the metabolic diseases associated with or expressed by renal
stone disease. The first thing we do is a complete work up of the patient to
discover the risk factors associated with calcium oxalate stone disease. For
instance, small diuresis, increased oxalate excretion, increased uric acid excretion, increased calcium excretion, or decreased citrate excretion. These are
some of the non-anatomical, metabolic risk factors associated with calcium
oxalate stone disease. Now, in the subgroup exhibiting increased uric acid
excretion, this abnormality could be due to two pathophysiological circum-
stances: metabolic uric acid overproduction and renal urate wasting. However, increased uric acid excretion is most commonly due to an exaggerated

consumption of purine-rich food. This hypothesis should be tested by placing the patient on a purine-free diet and retesting uric acid excretion. If he still excretes an increased amount of uric acid (say above 10 mg/kg of body weight per day), no matter what the serum urate level is, we treat him to decrease uric acid excretion. Now, how would I treat such a patient? I can recommend that he increase his daily water intake, but another wise treatment would be to prescribe allopurinol.

WATTS:
Do you think that there is a group of patients with calcium oxalate stone disease and normal urinary urate excretion on the diet that they currently take or that you can persuade them to take and whose propensity to calcium oxalate stone formation can be reduced by diminishing the rate of urinary urate excretion? Does this justify the use of allopurinol?

PUIG:
I would not say so.

WATTS:
Do you think there are any patients who fall into this category?

PUIG:
I would not say that there are no patients, but I would not treat a patient with calcium oxalate stone disease and normal uric acid excretion. If uric acid excretion is normal, I cannot say that uric acid is a conditioning factor for his calcium oxalate stone disease. Once anatomical abnormalities are excluded, I would look for one of the other risk factors that have already been mentioned and shown to be associated with calcium oxalate stone disease.

WATTS:
Does anybody else have a view on this subject? Well, if there is no further discussion on that point let us come back to something that has been more fully thought about over in the last days, namely, the question of whether to control the serum and urine uric acid because I think this is neglected material. This was the great throw-away source of information about patients' urine. Does controlling the serum and the urine uric acid levels protect the kidney? Should we treat the hyperuricemia in hyperuric acid patients with allopurinol to protect the kidneys?

SIMMONDS:
I wish to remind you of the data I showed yesterday, which compared results over the last 10 years in two young women who had presented with a single attack of gout. One is a carrier for PRPS superactivity and a uric acid overproducer, the other a young women with familial renal disease, who had been treated only for this. The PRPS carrier was treated only with colchicine.

She has never been given a uric acid lowering agent and despite persistent hyperuricaemia and hyperuricosuria, as far as we can measure her renal function is still fine. At the other end of the scale we have the young woman from one of these familial juvenile gouty nephropathy families (and there are many now) with hyperuricemia associated with renal urate hypoexcretion, also untreated for hyperuricemia, who progressed to dialysis and transplantation in the same time.

Numerous members of the latter kindreds have been treated for up to 20 years with allopurinol and their renal function has, in the majority, remained relatively stable. This is in contrast with the rapid decline in renal function in the above woman and that of the fathers, mothers, aunts and uncles in earlier generations of many kindreds with chis dominant disorder, sometimes affecting as many as five members, which, treated only for renal disease, led to death in the 1930's. As you know, if renal function is severely compromised at diagnosis and there is also hypertension, then despite allopurinol therapy it is likely that such cases will progress to dialysis and transplantation, but these are very rare. Consequently, in view of our experience at Guy's, we believe there is a strong reason for treating asymptomatic hyperuricemia in kindreds with familial juvenile gouty atrophy. Whether or not there is evidence of renal disease.

SIMMONDS:
One of our patients has had one single attack of gout and she was only treated with Colchicum, she has never been given any uric acid lowering agent and as far as we can measure her renal function she is still fine and as i said she has had no problem with a single attack of gout. So that is a situation of over-production of high plasma and urinary uric acid. There are many families now where you have this combination of the familiar juvenile gouty necropathy where certainly numerous members of the kindred would have had been treated with Allopurinol and where the renal function the rap of the clime has led to the death in the 30ies of their fathers, mothers, aunts, and uncles, and some times five members of the single kindred in the previous generation. These people are predominant to be still alive and their renal function, unless at the time they went on as you know, it was already severely compromised. Some of them went on to hypertension and renal insufficiency, they are declined to dyalysis and transplantation. So, that is in our opinion at Guy's Hospital is a case for treating even the asymptomatic members of a hyperuricacidaemia in those families who have no evidence of renal disease.

WATTS:
That is interesting because in the untreated state their uric acid excretion rate will not be raised because they are reabsorbing it.

SIMMONDS:
Yes, that is right.

WATTS:

So, you have got an increased circulation of uric acid within the kidney there all the time. Higher concentrations, particularly higher concentrations in the interstitial tissue of the kidney. And, whereas in your PRPP mutant that patient of course is excreating an uric acid liquid of the time is not recirculating to the kidney. I think that is a very interesting concept because one has tended to think perhaps the uric acid was in the urine was the thing which was the damaging to the kidney, but in fact is the uric acid recirculating within the kidney.

ZÖLLNER:

I do not want to discuss the rarities but the general case. In nearly all cases uric acid excretion reflects purine intake. Under experimental conditions one can manipulate uric acid excretion by manipulating dietary purines at will. You can even predict what will occur and, therefore, I think the determination of urinary uric acid is a very important factor in advising therapy because basically, and I come back to that point, therapy should involve dietary advice. With respect to the kidney I would like to point out that the urate concentration in the tissues of the kidney is the combined effect of urate in the plasma and in interstitial fluid. So, I think when we try to consider the kidney we must consider those complex correlations.

The point I wanted to make is that increased urinary uric acid excretion reflects over-production, but only in a very, very small part of patients of endogenous overproduction and in the vast majority of cases the production of uric acid from dietary purins.

WATTS:

So your message is that it is as important to measure urine uric acid as to measure blood uric acid.

EMMERSON:

I would like to refer back to the original question about whether controlling the urinary uric acid concentration is important in protecting the kidney. Our observations suggest that, in the absence of severe hyperuricaemia, a high urinary uric acid concentration is one of the factors potentially important in preventing uric acid induced renal disease. Indeed, it seems that, when allopurinol is administered, it may be the reduction in the urinary uric acid, as well as the serum uric acid, which has made uric acid nephropathy a much less common problem now than it used to be.

In relation to asymptomatic hyperuricaemia, I would like to suggest that controlling the hyperuricaemia does not necessarily involve the administration of drugs. We have found that determination of the factors contributing to the hyperuricaemia (such as excessive purine or regular alcohol consumption, obesity, hypertension or a suboptimal urine volume) can lead to a normalisation of hyperuricaemia if these factors can be corrected.

WATTS:
Yes, I think there has been a tendency to ignore it in the last 15 or 20 years.

NUKI:
I think this total advice is terribly an academic advice when you actually consider the scale of the community problem. Do we have any justification, telling general practitions that every time they pick up a raised plasma urate in a patient that they are investigating for something else, that they really have to do metabolic investigations to see whether this person is persistently hyperuricacidaemia? Let me put the question the other way round. With the exception of the families that we know of who have primary purine over-production because of inborn errors of metabolism, can frequently persent with renal problems and run into serious renal difficulties, I mean with the exception of the few but invisibly increasing number of families of the kind that Anne has described, we know of a single instance of a patient who has the common form of hyperuricacidaemia which is due to a difficulty in increasing a fractional excretion of urate in response to urate load. Do we have any single instance of knowledge of somebody like that who has had progressive problems of renal insufficiency without having concomitant symptomatic gout.

EMMERSON:
My comments related to the management of the hyperuricaemia in patients with gout and that we had not yet begun a consideration of asymptomatic hyperuricaemia.

WATTS:
Asymptomatic hyperuricacidaemia is going to come later on in the discussion, but I think George's point surely was the question whether one needs to be measuring urine uric acid as often as Prof. Zöllner was suggesting.

ZÖLLNER:
Yes, I would like to say one thing. The number of patients who have some sort of stone problems, no colics but possibly have a little blood in the urine, is large. We once studied 100 consecutive cases of urate nephrolithiasis from the urology department and in the majority of he patients urate levels had not been determined, urate excretion had not been measured.

SIMMONDS:
I would like to support Richard when he says that urine uric acid should also be measured. Moreover, I would like to suggest that gout in a young person is always unusual and is an indication for a detailed metabolic work-up, including urine uric acid levels. Only then can you find out whether they have a metabolic disorder resulting in uric acid overproduction, or hyperuricaemia due to renal urate hypoexcretion. In many instances general practitioners quite overlook these possibilities.

There is the example of two brothers who developed gout at 18 and 20 and were not investigated further but simply put on allopurinol up to 900 mg per day. They were referred to us via a neurologist at 46 and 48 when we diagnosed partial HGPRT deficiency. One of therm had no uric acid measurable in his urine whatsoever, it was all mostly xanthine and some hypoxanthine. At this point in time both brothers had a GFR of only 50 (although this had certainly been normal at original presentation), which we attributed to xanthine nephropathy, associated with the extremely high plasma and urine xanthine levels. This underlines another point I would like to make; namely that the allopurinol dose must always be adjusted carefully to avoid this, because subjects with HGPRT deficiency are peculiarly sensitive to allopurinol and plasma and urine xanthine and uric acid should be measured frequently.

WATTS:
One needs to know the serum uric acid concentration and the urinary urate excretion-rate when the patient is taking his own self-selected diet as well as when he is on a purine-free diet. This identifies patients with a high uric acid excretion that may be either dietary or due to one of the rare in-born errors of metabolism which accelerate purine *de novo* synthesis. If the urinary uric acid excretion is extremely high on the self-selected diet it may be necessary to repeat the study on a strict-purine-free diet if a genetic cause is suspected. That is to say, a genetic cause for urate over-production and over-excretion as opposed to the situation in autosomal dominant gout where there is a renal transport defect which reduces active tubular excretion.

EMMERSON:
It is our practice to undertake this as a routine in all of our gouty patients. We measure the urinary urate and creatinine excretion on their normal diet and again after a week on the low purine diet. This also documents their renal function (as the creatinine clearance) and enables one to calculate the urate clearance. It will also reveal the extent to which their usual purine and alcohol consumption is contributing to the serum urate and urinary urate excretion.

It is often said that these measurements are a very complex procedure when the underlying condition could be treated so simply with allopurinol without any investigation. However, my reply would be that, if you are thinking of treatment with a drug, you are probably going to be committed to a 20 year course of treatment and the cost of measuring the urine urate, in comparison with the commitment to a period of years of drug treatment, is infinitessimally small by comparison and even small by comparison with almost any other radiological or laboratory investigational procedure. Moreover, if you are planning to commit the patient to a long period of drug management, you should at least know the underlying problem you are dealing with and determine the factors contributing to it. One can readily determine from the history, examination and these investigations the factors which are contributing to the hyperuricaemia. Sometimes the patient can correct these, and we have had patients who became normouricaemic after correcting factors such as obesity and a poor urine volume. Although initially, the physician may need to commence drug treatment to prevent recurrent attacks of gout, it may well be possible to terminate drug treatment when the patient has been able to correct the cause and, in these cases, the withdrawal of treatment is possible because the cause is no longer operating. Since there are numerous correctable causes for hyperuricaemia, I believe one should investigate the patient to define these initially, even though some patients need to be treated with drugs in the short term.

WATTS:
I think so. Really our conclusion is that controlling the serum and urine uric acid level does in fact protect the kidney.

PUIG:
I would like to make some brief comments. First of all, uric acid is a potentially dangerous metabolic end product whose, fortunately, renal clearance can be measured. Let me make a parallelism with serum cholesterol, of which nowadays almost everybody knows his own level. We cannot measure urinary cholesterol, as cholesterol is not cleared by the kidney, but if we could we would certainly measure it. Why should we determine urinary uric acid excretion? As I pointed out yesterday, it is not easy to raise serum urate levels in a normal person. The normal kidney clears the excess uric acid from the body in a very efficient way. So in most patients, hyperuricemia means that there is a kidney impairment in clearing uric acid. Thus, it is good to look at urinary uric acid excretion. By the way, we simultaneously and always determine urinary creatinine excretion to assess the completeness of a given 24-hour urinary collection. By measuring urinary uric acid we examine what Dr Watts just pointed out: the individual production and/or intake of purines with a self-selected diet. If the patient underexcretes uric acid he may be diagnosed as having hyperuricemia with a proportionally low uric acid output. In such cases we do not reexamine the patient on a low-purine diet. But if the patient shows hyperuricemia with an increased uric acid output he could be an uric acid overproducer or he could have great fun from purine-rich food. In these cases, we believe that a reexamination on a purine-free diet is mandatory.

WATTS:
Yes.

PUIG:
The third comment I would like to make is related to hyperuricemia-induced kidney damage. Well, I think that several studies were carried out by Yü and Berger to address this question. They retrospectively analyzed an extensive

gouty population and divided it into two groups: one that received hypouricemic therapy and one who did not receive hypouricamic therapy. After a mean of 11 years, the inulin clearance was similar in both groups. This is one of the main arguments for saying that hyperuricemia per se does not damage the kidney and that asymptomatic hyperuricemia should not be treated. I believe that treatment of gouty hyperuricemia does protect some other parts of the body, but not the kidney.

EMMERSON:
The particular study which you quote was a retrospective look at data from a group of gouty patients and was not designed to answer the question you pose. I do not believe that it enables one to draw the conclusions you have expressed.

PUIG:
The other studies were an expansion of previous studies by Yü and Berger comprising 624 patients with gout. By dividing these patients into different groups and performing variance analysis, the authors concluded that the strongest correlate for decreased inulin clearance in their gouty population was hypertension, ischemic heart disease, and preexisting chronic renal diseases, such as glomerulonephritis, infectious pyelonephritis or amyloidosis. In addition, in a controlled study Fessel et al observed that after a mean interval of 8 years, azotemia developed in 1.8% of asymptomatic hyperuricemic patients and in 2.1% of normouricemic controls. From these studies we may conclude that asymptomatic hyperuricemia is unlikely to lead to serious renal insufficiency and thus should not be treated. In patients with gout, the development of renal insufficiency should be attributed to a complicating condition sich as hypertension or atherosclerosis.

EMMERSON:
I do not believe that this interpretation gives the overall picture relating to this problem since it is looking at a situation which has changed since the advent of allopurinol treatment. While admitting that patients whose gout is well treated do not now develop progressive renal damage and that gouty nephropathy is now an uncommon disorder, this does not mean that gouty renal disease did not often occur or cannot still occur if therapy is inadequate. Currently, it is rarely seen because most gout is well treated and nephropathy does not develop.

I would also disagree with yout statement that the consumption of purines does not cause an elevation of the serum urate concentration in normal persons. It will certainly do so since I have observed it on myself and it has been frequently demonstrated that consumption of a purine containing diet in normal persons will cause any elevation of the serum urate concentration.

NUKI:
I think we don't think we can answer the question. If we really believe that there is a hypothesis that prolonged asymptomatic hyperuricacidaemia or hyperuricaciduria is associated with progressive renal loss of renal function we have to show that we can prevent it by treating it in a proper perspective control trial and until we do that I don't think any amount of having people sitting around tables saying what their opinion is, will make any difference.

GRÖBNER:
During the 3rd International Symposium on purine metabolism in man in 1979 Diez et al. presented a paper concerning the natural course of gout. They have studied the mortality rate and evolution of gout disease in 125 patients with a 10 year follow up. Of 53 deaths 18 were due to renal failure; that means at least 33% of all patients had renal problems.

SIMMONDS:
There was a study that Terry Gibson did at Guy's Hospital. For two years he studied a comparable group of gouty patients, half of them were on Colchicum, and half of them were on Allopurinol, and really there was no significant difference in their GFR in the two groups at the end of that two-years' period.

WATTS:
But two years is awfully short.

SIMMONDS:
I know, but this is the only such study I am aware of.

ZÖLLNER:
I think it was very pertinent by George Nuki to quote those hypertension ideas and studies. I would like to quote a study from Chicago where the epidemiologist studied a prognosis of obesity over five years in men who were below the age of 50 and not unexpectedly, it was found that these obese people have a better life expectancy in a five-year's period than those who have lost weight. But never they woul doubt the data from the statistics of the life insurances that in general obese people live shorter. Results depend on the length of the study. In the case of hyperuricemia one couldn't get the permission for such a long study in this country. We have a question which we must answer by the best guess, which cannot be answered by a prospective study.

SCOTT:
May I came in here, because Anne has in fact misquoted Terry Gibson's study. Terry Gibson studied a Colchicine-treated group and an Allopurinol treated group of gout patients and found that the rise in plasma creatinine which took place in the colchicine group did not take place in the Allopurinol-

treated group. The trouble with this study is that the plasma creatinine in the two groups was different when he started the study. This is what the statisticians call a deviation towards the mean.

. . . These patients should be thoroughly investigated, but it is rarely necessary to treat them, apart from patients with kidney disease, a different category. Twenty years ago I identified a young man with gout, an over-producer with deficiency of HGPRT. His younger brother of twelve was quite well, but he had the same enzyme defect. This younger brother has been swallowing allopurinol for twenty years, which I think is justified because of the well-documented risk of gout and kidney stones.

PUIG:
As I mentioned in the discussion of Dr Scott's paper we should look for any deposition of urate in a patient with hyperuricemia. We don't usually order a complete X-ray study on every asymptomatic hyperuricemic patient. So, when can we confidently say that hyperuricemia had no consequences in a patient? I wouldn't treat most asymptomatic hyperuricemic patients, but yesterday in discussing the comments by Anne Simmonds I said that I treated a 12-year-old young lady with allopurinol. This lady has a familial nephropathy with asymptomatic hyperuricemia, and I would have done the same as Dr Scott did if the patient had HPRT deficiency. For the general population with asymptomatic hyperuricemia I would not use uric acid lowering agents, but in special conditons such as HPRT deficiency, PRPPs overactivity or familial disorders, I would probably use allopurinol.

WATTS:
Can we say the threshold level above which patients should or would or should not betreated. This takes us back, to my knowledge, almost 20 years. Who would like to answer this question?

EMMERSON:
Yes, the studies of Fessel and others have shown that there is little risk of developing renal pathology in persons with serum urates of up to 13 mg per cent, that is, about 0.7 mmol per litre. The evidence for this seems good and we must accept it as the best available currently. On the other hand, most people with asymptomatic hyperuricaemia have serum urate concentrations of less than 0.6 mmol per litre. This causes me little concern and, at this level, I am happy to leave them untreated. However, I confess to being a little concerned if the serum urate is persistently above this level, although it is rare that asymptomatic hyperuricaemia of this degree is seen to be persistent.

On the other hand, I do not believe that any wish to lower the serum urate is necessarily a commitment to drug treatment. While following the serum urate concentration in a patient with asymptomatic hyperuricaemia, we should be defining the cause in that individual and correcting the causes where possible. Rather than prescribing 20 years of drug treatment, we should ensure that the causes are investigated and corrected. When approached in this way, there will be very few patients whose hyperuricaemia is persistently greater than 0.6 mmol per litre. After many years of observation, we have not observed the development of renal problems in patients with hyperuricaemia of this degree, although the higher the serum urate concentration, the greater the risk of developing gouty arthritis. I do believe that, particularly in the management of asymptomatic hyperuricaemia, it is important to approach the cause rather than accepting that drug treatment will be necessary.

SCOTT:
. . . The ease with which you can investigate a case of hyperuricaemia depends very much on the patient. In the case of a young person you can talk to the patient and his parents and they will readily agree to a low purine diet so that adequate investigations will be done. But in no way will you get an obese alcoholic man of 70 on a low purine diet, and it wouldn't worry me very much.

WATTS:
And still less you are going to get him onto a low-purin diet for the rest of his life.

ZÖLLNER:
Certainly, this is the case with diet. But consider a person who will not take his diet. Or wouldn't this just be a case for drug therapy? In my mind it would.

EMMERSON:
In relation to showing that lifestyle modification can lead to lowering of the serum urate concentration, I think it will be almost impossible to acquire a sufficiently large group of patients to be able to prove its value statistically. However, we can all see it happen in individual patients who are prepared to modify their lifestyle to observe the effect it can have on their serum urate concentration.

I would also like to comment on what has been said of a low purine diet. In our practice, a low purine diet is principally an investigational tool and is never a treatment option. However, in saying that, it is important to realize that many hyperuricaemic patients actually take a high purine diet whereas a moderate purine diet may in fact seem like a low purine diet to them. It is relatively easy for many patients to have a normal purine diet rather than a high purine diet but a true low purine diet is rarely a long-term therapeutic alternative.

SCOTT:
And what about a low-calorie diet?

EMMERSON:
There are people in whom a low calorie diet can restore body weight to normal, which can result in restoration of a normal serum urate. However, many of these people find it difficult to remain permanently on a low calorie diet. When they gain weight again, their hyperuricaemia returns.

SCOTT:
And what about uric acid?

WATTS:
So, as the people now feel we should treat patients of asymptomatic hyperuricacidaemia with drugs if we can't modify their lifestyle.

ZÖLLNER:
Well we still have to discuss what border level . . . I certainly would never treat a patient with levels below 7.5 mg/l with a drug. If a patient produces tophi, particularly in unusual or even dangerous places, you cannot say "I wont give you the drug". You should discuss the case with the patient. It is basically – and this is my believe – a question you must work out together with the patient.

NUKI:
That is only you say that with plasma uric acid level of 10 you have a very high risk of getting calculi, that was originally based, as far as I remember, Framingham studies, larger population studies, when they studied more than 2000 men over, I think it was 10 or 12 years, and although they found, I think it was 9 men who had calculi, those calculi were never established with any kind of stone lysis or anything. I just wonder how high the risk is.

EMMERSON:
The risk of gout at a serum urate of 0.54 mmol per litre has been calculated from population studies as being about 5 per cent per annum – that is, there is an annual risk of one in twenty hyperuricaemic patients developing gout in any one year. On the other hand, the risk of patients with asymptomatic hyperuricaemia developing renal calculi is much lower than the risk of gout, being less than half a per cent per annum.

Subject Index